# TRANSFUSION MEDICINE AND SCIENTIFIC DEVELOPMENTS

Edited by **A.W.M.M. Koopman-van Gemert**

**Transfusion Medicine and Scientific Developments**
http://dx.doi.org/10.5772/66265
Edited by A.W.M.M. Koopman-van Gemert

**Contributors**

Xingshun Qi, Fernando Romeiro, Yiling Li, Xingbin Hu, Jinmei Xu, Mark D. Scott, Wendy Toyofuku, Xining Yang, Meera Raj, Ning Kang, Rajiv Saxena, Eren Arslan Davulcu, Fahri Sahin, Guray Saydam, Anil Tombak, Deqing Wang, Leiying Zhang

**Published by InTech**
Janeza Trdine 9, 51000 Rijeka, Croatia



**Publishing Process Manager** Dajana Pemac
**Technical Editor** SPi Global
**Cover** InTech Design team

First published July, 2017
Printed in Croatia
Legal deposit, Croatia: National and University Library in Zagreb

Additional hard copies can be obtained from orders@intechopen.com

Transfusion Medicine and Scientific Developments, Edited by A.W.M.M. Koopman-van Gemert
p. cm.
Print ISBN 978-953-51-3319-3
Online ISBN 978-953-51-3320-9

For EU product safety concerns:
IN TECH d.o.o., Prolaz Marije Krucifikse Kozulić 3, 51000 Rijeka, Croatia, info@intechopen.com or visit our website at intechopen.com.

# Meet the editor

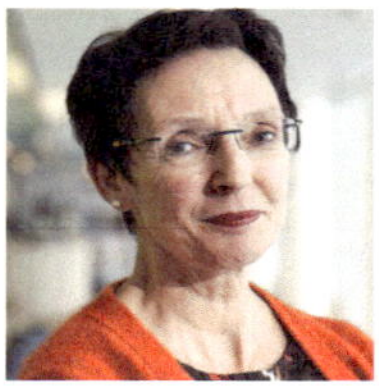

Dr. Anna Wilhelmina Margaretha Maria Koopman-van Gemert MD, PhD, became anaesthesiologist-intensivist from the Radboud University Nijmegen (the Netherlands) in 1987. She worked for a couple of years also as a blood bank director in Nijmegen and introduced in the Netherlands the Cell Saver and blood transfusion alternatives. She performed research in perioperative autotransfusion and obtained the degree of PhD in 1993 publishing *Peri-operative autotransfusion by means of a blood cell separator*.
Blood transfusion had her special interest being the president of the Haemovigilance Chamber TRIP and performing several tasks in local and national blood bank and anticoagulant-blood transfusion guidelines committees. Currently, she is working as an associate professor and up till recently was the dean at the Albert Schweitzer Hospital Dordrecht. She performed (inter)national tasks as vice-president of the Concilium Anaesthesia and related committees.
She performed research in several fields, with over 100 publications in (inter)national journals and numerous papers on scientific conferences. She received several awards and is a member of Honour of the Dutch Society of Anaesthesia.

# Contents

# Preface

The function of the human blood remains a fascinating subject, and research is extensively performed to explain all its functions and pathology. In 1818, James Blundell, an obstetrician, was generally considered as being the first person to perform a blood transfusion using homologous blood. At that moment, the blood group system was unknown until Karl Landsteiner distinguished it in 1901. After that, the possibility and safety of homologous and autologous blood transfusion were investigated and became possible. At that moment, blood transfusion has become an integral part of clinical practice.

Blood transfusion has become over the last decades a tremendously important field of research. The knowledge of this complicated science increased, and relations, not known before, were discovered, such as the importance of prevention of antibody formation during blood transfusion, a part of the mechanism behind trauma-related coagulopathy, the role of the glycocalyx and the importance and besides plasma's coagulation repairing function, the probability of plasma-restoring properties of the glycocalyx in the transfusion cascade. Also the knowledge about the broader function of the red blood cells, not only being an oxygen-transporting medium, has grown. The same is true for platelets and the clotting factors.

In the recent years, the technological developments have introduced a sophisticated blood bank service, performing scientific research as well. Transfusion medicine has become a specialization, including immunology, haematology, microbiology, development of alternatives and improving perioperative transfusion therapy.

This book is not a textbook about transfusion medicine and is not meant to cover all subjects related to transfusion. Instead, several, often unknown, aspects of blood cells and transfusion strategies are discussed. Subjects in this book are immunological and span aspects of red blood cells and their function in thrombosis. The specific, often not known, role of platelets in inflammation is discussed. Attention is also on several indications for blood transfusion such as functional dose of red blood cells, transfusion strategies in gastrointestinal bleedings and transplantation surgery.

We hope this book will provide readers with more knowledge about blood components and blood transfusion, applicable in clinical practice.

I want to thank the authors for the extensive job they have performed and their excellent contribution to this book. I am thankful to the publishing process manager, Ms. Dajana Pemac, who has excellently performed the compilation of this book with dedicated care.

**Dr. A.W.M.M. Koopman-van Gemert, MD, PhD**
Department of Anaesthesiology
Albert Schweitzer Hospital, Dordrecht
The Netherlands

Section 1

# Immunomodulatory Properties of Red Blood Cells

Chapter 1

# A Double *In Vivo* Biotinylation Technique to Assess Erythrocyte Turnover in Blood Circulation

Sreoshi Chatterjee and Rajiv K. Saxena

Additional information is available at the end of the chapter

http://dx.doi.org/10.5772/intechopen.69133

**Abstract**

We have developed a new double *in vivo* biotinylation (DIB) technique that may be used for assessing turnover patterns of erythrocytes in circulation. This technique involves two successive *in vivo* biotinylation steps, interspersed by a period of 5–30 days, which would enable us to tag with biotin a population of erythrocytes entering blood circulation over a defined period of time, between the two biotinylation steps. As such we can track the age-related changes in a lifetime of the circulating erythrocytes, or we can simultaneously study two defined age cohorts of aged as well as young erythrocytes in circulation. We have extensively used this technique to look at erythrocyte loss in mouse models of anemia induced by (a) heavy metal cadmium (Cd), (b) herbicide Paraquat (PQ), (c) carbon nanotubes (CNTs), and (d) autoantibody in autoimmune hemolytic anemia (AIHA). We have found that the pattern of erythrocyte removal is distinctly different in different models of murine anemia. In certain types of anemia (CNT and AIHA), younger erythrocytes in blood circulation are preferentially removed, whereas in other cases (Cd and PQ), old erythrocytes are specifically eliminated.

**Keywords:** DIB technique, flow cytometry, erythrocyte turnover, anemia, mouse models of anemia, cadmium, Paraquat, carbon nanotubes, autoantibody, AIHA

## 1. Introduction

Erythrocytes constitute almost 99.9% of all blood cells, excluding platelets. Erythrocytes have a definite lifespan in the circulation during which time they shuttle through the entire body several times exchanging respiratory gases between tissues and organs. The lifespan of human and murine erythrocytes has been estimated to be around 120 and 50 days, respectively, indicating that roughly 1% of all circulating erythrocytes in human and 2% in mice are destroyed each day [1–3]. Erythrocytes undergo repetitive cycles of oxidation and reduction during gaseous exchange, are regularly exposed to severe osmotic shock while passing through the kidney medulla, and have to squeeze through very narrow blood capillaries. As the erythrocytes age in circulation, these repeated insults result in accumulation of several changes in the cell, particularly in the membrane composition. These damaged erythrocytes are prone to destruction in the reticuloendothelial system (RES) in the spleen, bone marrow, and liver [4].

Studies in the past have aimed to decipher the actual kinetics of erythrocyte turnover in circulation, but their approaches have been marred by the unavailability of a suitable technique to identify erythrocytes of different age groups. Mostly they have relied upon buoyant density of the erythrocytes [5, 6] or hyper-transfusion studies [7]. Later with the advent of biotinylation studies [8–10], things became clearer, and finally with the novel double *in vivo* biotinylation (DIB) technique developed in our lab [11, 12], we have now been able to solve the mystery of the kinetics of erythrocyte survival in the blood [11–16]. Studies on erythrocyte survival kinetics and the associated age-related changes in buoyant density, autofluorescence, and phosphatidylserine (PS) externalization have extensively been reviewed in Saxena et al. [16].

Using the DIB technique, erythrocyte turnover kinetics in a normal murine system is now well understood. However in the case of anemia, where the homeostasis between erythrocyte destruction and erythropoiesis is disturbed, the erythrocyte turnover pattern may completely alter. To understand the fate of erythrocyte turnover in conditions of anemia, we studied four mouse models of experimental anemia, namely anemia induced by (a) toxic heavy metal cadmium (Cd) ions [17], (b) herbicide Paraquat (PQ) [18], (c) carbon nanotubes (CNTs) [19], and (d) autoantibody in autoimmune hemolytic anemia (AIHA) [20].

## 2. The double *in vivo* biotinylation (DIB) technique

Advent of the DIB technique, recently developed in our laboratory, has made it possible to simultaneously enumerate and study erythrocytes of different age groups in blood circulation [11, 12, 16]. In the DIB protocol, circulating erythrocytes were biotinylated in two steps by intravenous administration of biotin-X-N-hydroxysuccinimide ester (BXN), through the tail vein of mice. The first step of high-intensity biotinylation involved three daily intravenous (*i.v.*) injections of biotin (1 mg), followed after few days by a low-intensity biotin injection with a single lower dose (0.6 mg). The first step labels all the erythrocytes present in circulation at the time of injection, while the second step labels the fresh erythrocytes that were released in circulation in the period between the two biotinylation steps. At any time point after the second biotinylation, biotin intensity on circulating erythrocytes could be analyzed by flow cytometry after staining the erythrocytes with streptavidin coupled to an appropriate fluorochrome [11, 12, 16]. As such erythrocytes in circulation could be grouped into three distinct cohorts: (i) biotin$^{negative}$ erythrocytes that represents the fresh erythrocytes that were released in the blood after the second step of biotinylation, (ii) biotin$^{low}$ erythrocytes that consists of the cohort of erythrocytes released in the blood between the two steps of biotinylation, and (iii) biotin$^{high}$ erythrocytes that comprise the residual erythrocytes from the ones that were present in circulation at the time of the first biotinylation step [16]. The DIB protocol has been summarized in **Figure 1**.

Time interval between the two biotin injections can be altered according to the requirement of the experiment [16]. In DIB protocol A, a window of 5 days is provided between the two steps. This enables us to track the circulating erythrocytes from the moment of its release into the bloodstream till the end of its lifespan. Alternatively by introducing a long gap (of about 30 days) in DIB protocol B, two defined cohorts of aged as well as young erythrocytes in circulation can be identified and studied simultaneously. For details, see **Figure 1**.

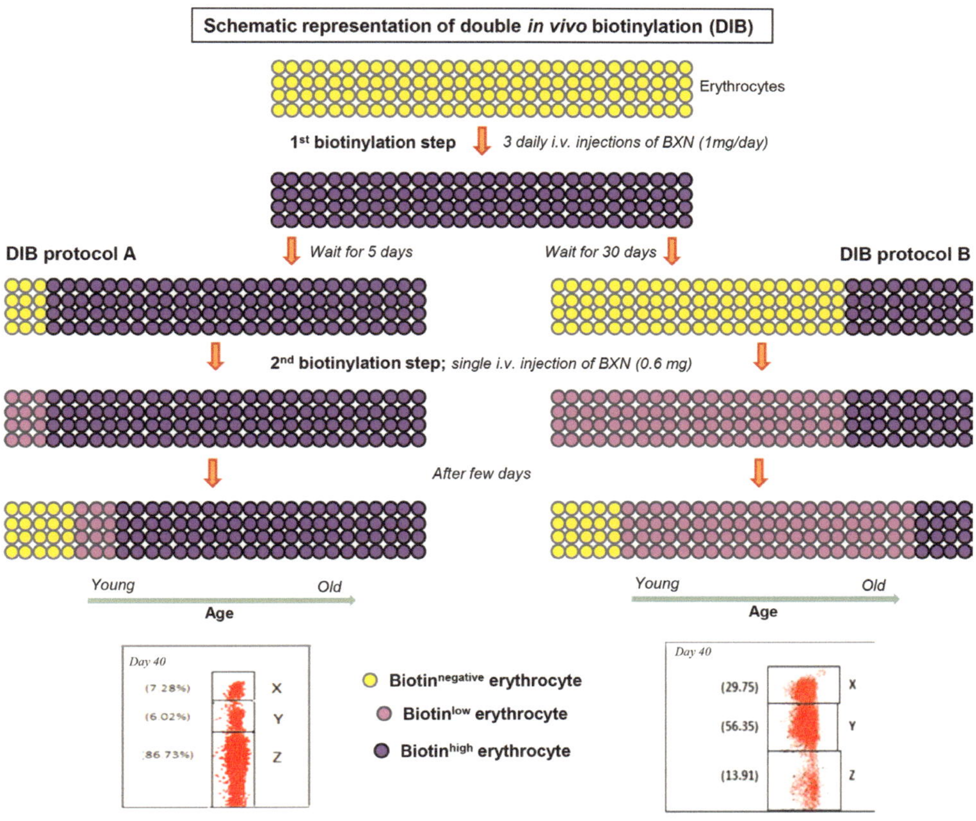


**Figure 1. Double *in vivo* biotinylation (DIB) technique**. C57BL/6 mice were given three daily *i.v.* doses of 1 mg BXN (first biotinylation step), followed, after a rest for several days, by a single additional dose of 0.6 mg BXN (second biotinylation step). Biotin label on erythrocytes was examined at different time points by bleeding the mice and staining the cells with streptavidin-APC followed by flow cytometry. In DIB protocol A, a window of 5 days is provided between the two biotinylation steps; in DIB protocol B, a long gap of 30 days is introduced. Principle of the technique and the residual biotin label on circulating erythrocytes are shown above. Erythrocyte populations in boxes X, Y, and Z represent biotin$^{high}$, biotin$^{low}$, and biotin$^{negative}$ erythrocytes, respectively; values in parentheses represent percentage of cells in different boxes.

# 3. Erythrocyte turnover in the blood

Erythrocytes have a definite lifespan in the circulation during which time they shuttle through the entire body several times exchanging respiratory gases between tissues and organs. Using the DIB technique, we have been able to follow the survival kinetics of a cohort of erythrocytes of defined age, with a degree of precision not possible so far. Based on this technique, Khandelwal and Saxena [11] described the triphasic nature of survival kinetics of blood erythrocytes in circulation. This profile has been depicted in **Figure 2**. In this system, a defined cohort of erythrocytes remained more or less constant till 10 days after their release in circulation and

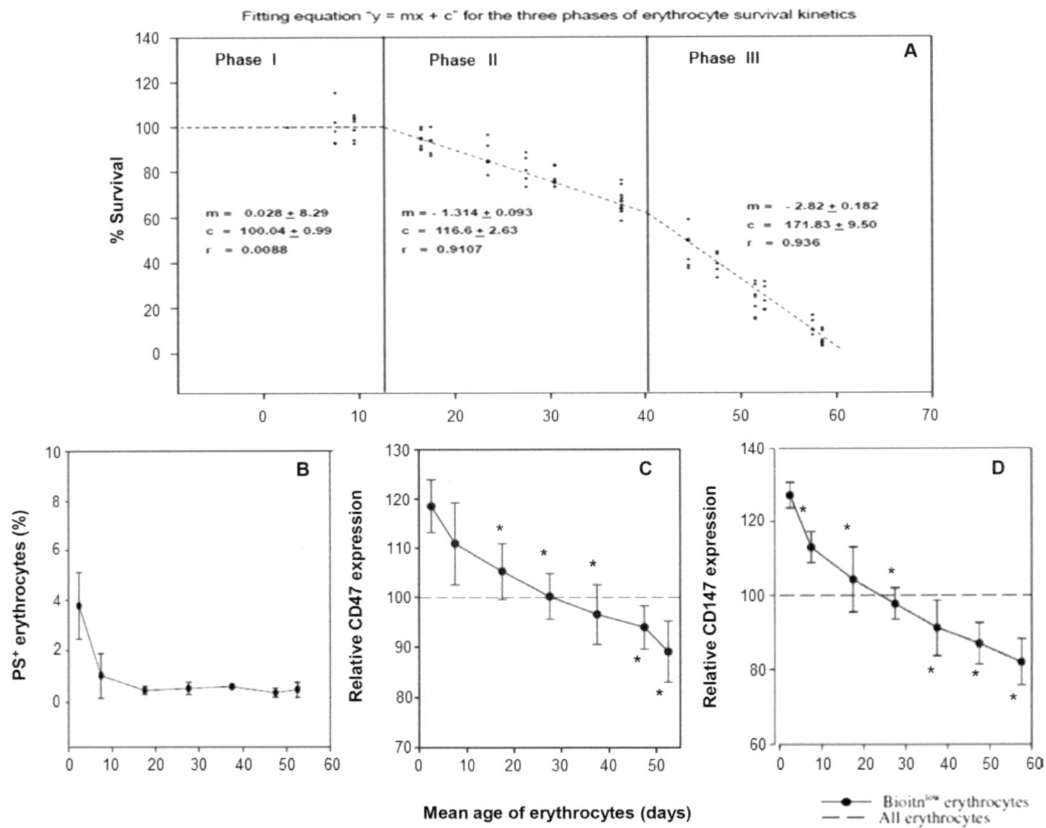


**Figure 2. Survival kinetics of erythrocytes in circulation.** C57BL/6 mice were DIB labeled following protocol A. At different time points, the biotin$^{low}$ population was assessed as percentage of all circulating erythrocytes and followed throughout their lifespan in the blood. Panel A shows the survival kinetics of murine erythrocytes. Correlation coefficients and slopes of the three phases of the decay curve have been calculated (n = 14). PS externalization and expression of CD47 and CD147 were studied on the biotin$^{low}$ population during its lifespan in the blood. Panel B shows the proportion of PS$^{+}$ erythrocytes. As compared to the first time point, the decline in PS expression on all subsequent time points was statistically significant. CD47 and CD147 expression are given in panels C and D, respectively. Mean CD47 and CD147 expression on the biotin$^{low}$ population has been expressed as percentage of the mean expression on all blood erythrocytes. Each point in the graph represents mean ± SD of observations. n = 5. $*p < 0.05$ for comparison of the groups. Statistical analysis was done using Student t-test.

started to decline constantly thereafter, indicating a random destruction irrespective of age. The rate of this decline increased after about 40 days in circulation, suggesting the onset of an age-dependent selective killing of erythrocytes [11, 15]. Thus the true picture of erythrocyte destruction in mice circulation appears to be a combination of both random killing, at least in the first segment of the life cycle, and the age-dependent destruction, especially in the latter part of the life span.

The factors that drive such unique survival kinetics of circulating erythrocytes are not clearly understood. The role of PS externalization might be critical in this respect. Annexin V staining of biotin$^{low}$ erythrocytes at different time points reveals that PS extrusion is more efficient in younger erythrocytes rather than in senescent ones (**Figure 2B**) [12]. It is likely that younger erythrocytes that get damaged due to oxidative or other forms of stress may readily extrude PS and undergo erythrophagocytosis, leading to random killing of erythrocytes. On the other hand, a steady fall in CD47 [14] and CD147 [11] expression has been observed during aging of erythrocytes (**Figure 2C** and **D**). These may render older erythrocytes susceptible to phagocytosis by macrophages.

## 4. Murine models of anemia

### 4.1. Cadmium (Cd)-induced anemia

Cadmium, one of the most toxic heavy metals, a category I carcinogen [21], is a nonbiodegradable environmental contaminant that can cause serious health hazard [21–24]. Exposure to cadmium may occur through contamination in food and drinking water [25], cigarette smoke [26, 27], or through occupational exposure in mining and manufacturing industries [23, 27, 28]. Cadmium has a long biological half-life of 10–30 years and can accumulate into various organs and tissues, particularly in kidneys [29] and also in the lung, liver, bone, testis, cardiovascular, and the immune systems, causing severe damage [29, 30]. Anemia as a consequence of cadmium toxicity has been observed in many cases of human exposure [31–33] and also in animal models [34–38].

In our experiment groups of mice were given 1000 ppm of cadmium chloride in drinking water, and their blood parameters were monitored every week. Continuous exposure to cadmium induced a significant decline in erythrocyte count and hemoglobin content, indicating anemia (**Figure 3**, panels A and B). A significant decline in blood parameters could be observed as early as in the second week of exposure [17]. Exposure to lower dose of cadmium (50 ppm $CdCl_2$) resulted in the development of a transient anemia in mice [17].

### 4.2. Herbicide Paraquat (PQ)-induced anemia

Paraquat (N, N′-dimethyl-4, 4′-bipyridinium dichloride, PQ), one of the most widely used herbicide, kills plants rapidly by deactivating the photosynthetic mechanism. It also has considerable toxicity toward animals and humans and has widely been used for suicide throughout the world [39–41]. Ingestion of PQ causes liver, lung, heart, and kidney failure within several

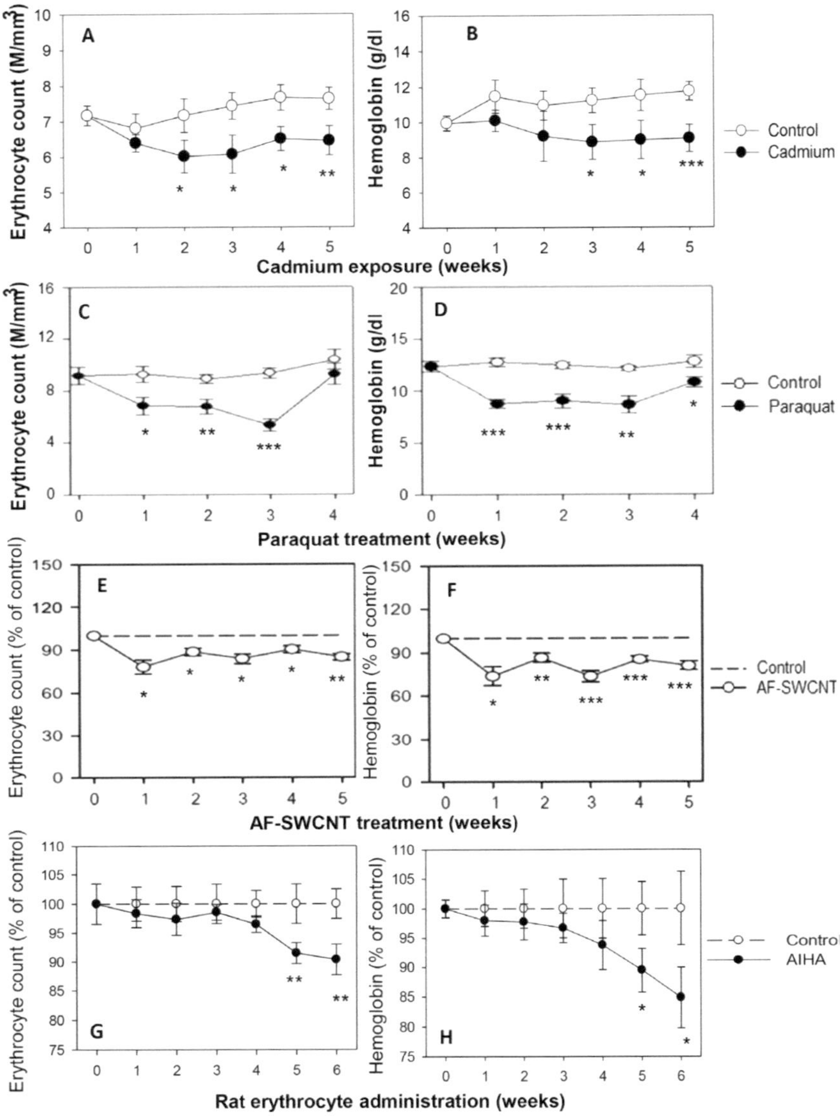


**Figure 3. Induction of anemia in mice.** Anemia was induced in mice through different stimuli. Blood samples from mice were collected at different time points and analyzed on an automated cell counter. Erythrocyte count and hemoglobin content in cadmium (Cd)-induced anemia (panels A and B), Paraquat (PQ)-induced anemia (panels C and D), carbon nanotube (CNT)-induced anemia (panels E and F), and autoimmune hemolytic anemia (AIHA, panels G and H) are shown above. Each point on the graph represents mean ±SEM of observations. n = 10. *$p < 0.05$, **$p < 0.01$, and ****$p < 0.001$ for comparison of the groups. Statistical analysis was done using Student t-test.

days to several weeks [42]. A link between the exposure to PQ and Parkinson's disease has also been reported [43]. PQ is a potent inducer of reactive oxygen species (ROS), and occurrence of anemia as a consequence of exposure to PQ has also been documented [44, 45]. The use of PQ was banned in Europe in 2007, but the herbicide is still widely used in the rest of the world.

In our experiment mice were administered repeated doses of Paraquat (Paraquat dichloride hydrate freshly dissolved in phosphate buffered saline (PBS), 10 mg/kg of body weight) intraperitoneally (*i.p.*) on alternate days [18, 43]. Control mice received vehicle alone. Blood parameters were monitored at different time points. Paraquat treatment induced a transient anemia in mice, indicated by a significant decline in blood erythrocyte count (up to 45%) as well as blood hemoglobin levels (upto 38%) on 7, 14, and 21 day time points (**Figure 3**, panels C and D) [18]. Erythrocyte count as well as blood hemoglobin levels however returned to normal by the end of 4 weeks, even though PQ treatment was continued.

### 4.3. Carbon nanotube (CNT)-induced anemia

Nanoparticles are defined as particulate dispersions or solid particles with a size in the range of 10–100 nm. Single-walled carbon nanotubes (SWCNTs) are a class of engineered nanomaterials that represent rolled-up tubes of graphite sheet of sp2 hybridized carbon atoms, having a diameter of about 1 nm. Due to their unique structural and remarkable electronic, mechanical, and chemical properties, engineered nanomaterials find wide applications in molecular electronics, microdevices, gas storage, catalytic supports, aerospace, automobile, and atomic force microscopy and biological applications like biosensors, drug delivery, etc. [46–48]. Interaction of nanoparticles with the body is dependent on their size, chemical composition, surface structure, solubility, and shape [49–51]. Several studies have demonstrated the toxicity of SWCNT to different types of cells *in vitro* [52–54] and *in vivo* [55–58].

In our experiment, mice were administrated *i.v.* 10 mg acid-functionalized SWCNTs (AF-SWCNTs) on alternate days, and blood parameters were examined at different time points. Significant decline in erythrocyte count as well as hemoglobin levels was observed at different time points during the treatment with AF-SWCNTs [19]. Results in **Figure 3**, panels E and F show that erythrocyte count and hemoglobin levels decreased by 10–22% and 13–25%, respectively, at different time points. Repeated administration of AF-SWCNTs (10 mg) induced a sustained anemia in mice [19].

### 4.4. Autoimmune hemolytic anemia (AIHA)

Autoimmune hemolytic anemia (AIHA) is characterized by the production of pathogenic self-reactive autoantibodies against self-erythrocytes that can result in premature destruction of erythrocytes leading to the clinical manifestation of anemia [59–62]. Pathogenesis of AIHA involves two underlying mechanisms, namely erythrophagocytosis of autoantibody-coated erythrocytes by macrophages in the reticuloendothelial system in the liver and spleen [63, 64] and complement-mediated lysis of erythrocytes following binding of IgM autoantibodies [65].

AIHA could be induced in mice following the Playfair and Clarke Model [66], based on Weigle's hypothesis of termination of immunological unresponsiveness to an antigen by injection of a cross-reacting antigen with similar/shared epitopes [67]. In this model repeated injection of rat erythrocytes induces production of autoantibodies against self-erythrocytes in mice [68–70]. The immunized mice develop autoimmune anemia, a severe but transient one, characterized by the presence of both anti-mouse autoantibody and the usual anti-rat antibody [69].

In our experiment mice were given weekly *i.p.* injections of $2 \times 10^8$ rat erythrocytes, and blood parameters were monitored at regular intervals. Generation of anti-mouse erythrocyte auto-antibody was estimated by flow cytometric analysis of erythrocytes stained with anti-mouse IgG/IgM-fluorescein isothiocyanate (FITC) polyclonal antibodies [71, 72]. The results show that a significant anemia was demonstrable in the immunized mice only after 5–6 weekly administrations of rat erythrocytes [20], when the blood erythrocyte count suffered a 10% decline and hemoglobin a staggering 15% decline (**Figure 3**, panels G and H, respectively). The anti-mouse erythrocyte autoantibody level also showed a sharp increase at the same time point [20], indicating an autoimmune response.

## 5. Erythrocyte turnover pattern in different models of anemia

Turnover profile for the various age cohorts of circulating erythrocytes was examined by utilizing the DIB technique of erythrocyte labeling *in vivo* to analyze the age-dependent susceptibility of circulating erythrocytes to the different mediators of stress, Cd, PQ, CNTs, and AIHA. Erythrocytes isolated from the peripheral blood of the DIB-labeled mice were stained *ex vivo* with streptavidin-allophycocyanin (APC) and anti-mouse CD71-PE followed by flow cytometry. Circulating erythrocytes were delineated as per the relative streptavidin and CD71 staining into four different groups: biotin$^{high}$ (older erythrocytes), biotin$^{low}$ (intermediate age group), CD71$^-$biotin$^{negative}$ (young) erythrocytes, and CD71$^+$biotin$^{negative}$ reticulocytes. A representative flow diagram is shown in **Figure 4**. A comparison of the proportion of erythrocytes

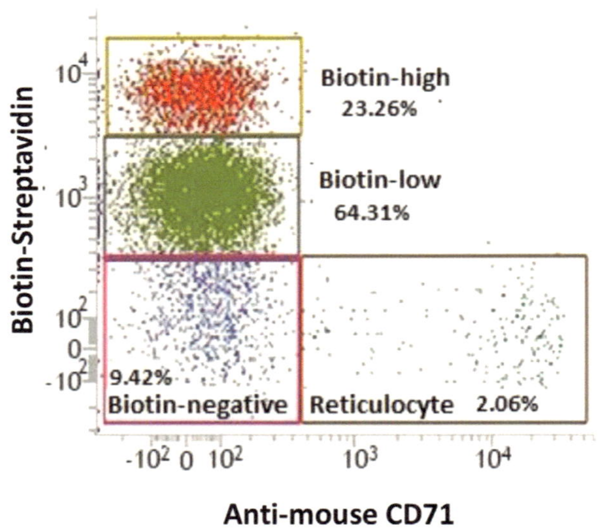


**Figure 4. Age cohorts of circulating erythrocytes**. Mouse erythrocytes were labeled with biotin *in vivo* by the two-step biotinylation procedure (DIB protocol B). Blood samples were collected, and erythrocytes were stained *ex vivo* with streptavidin-APC and anti-mouse CD71-PE. Proportions of the different age cohorts were determined as biotin$^{high}$ (older erythrocytes), biotin$^{low}$ (intermediate age group), CD71$^-$biotin$^{negative}$ (young erythrocytes), and CD71$^+$biotin$^{negative}$ reticulocytes. Representative flow histograms showing the proportion of different age groups of erythrocytes are shown.

http://dx.doi.org/10.5772/intechopen.69133

belonging to different age cohorts would give their turnover profile. Interestingly, results from the four models of murine anemia could be clustered into two distinct categories, with completely contrasting characters.

### 5.1. Increased susceptibility of older erythrocytes: Cd and PQ

Exposure to environmental toxicants cadmium and Paraquat resulted in a very similar response in terms of erythrocyte turnover. The turnover profiles indicate that the kinetics of decline of older erythrocytes (biotin$^{high}$ subpopulations that entered blood circulation before the first biotinylation step; **Figure 5**, panels A and B) and the increase in the proportion of younger subpopulation of erythrocytes (biotin$^{negative}$, entering blood circulation after the second biotinylation step; **Figure 5**, panels C and D) was significantly higher in the treatment groups than the control (**Figure 5**) [17, 18]. These results suggest that the older erythrocytes in blood circulation may be preferentially eliminated in the toxicant (Cd or PQ)-exposed mice, leaving the young

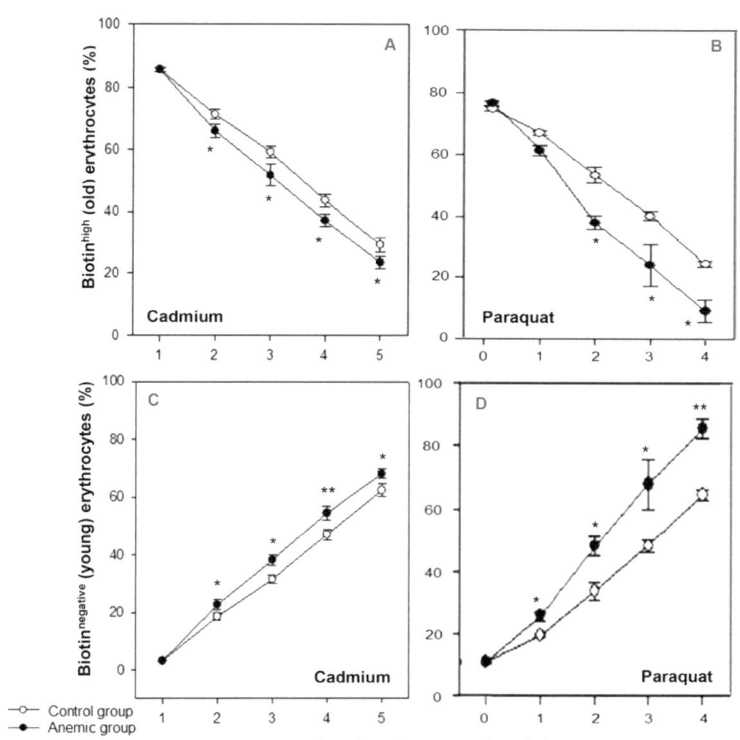


**Figure 5. Erythrocyte turnover in the blood of mice exposed to cadmium and Paraquat.** Mice were rendered anemic by exposure to toxicants like cadmium and Paraquat. Mouse erythrocytes were labeled with biotin *in vivo* by the two-step biotinylation procedure (protocol A). Erythrocytes were stained *ex vivo* with streptavidin-APC, and proportions of the different age cohorts were determined. Turnover profile of relatively aged biotin$^{high}$ (panels A and B) and young biotin$^{negative}$ (panels C and D) erythrocytes in cadmium-treated (panels A and C) and Paraquat-treated (panels B and D) mice has been shown above. Each point on the graph represents mean ±SEM of observations. n = 10. *$p < 0.05$ and **$p < 0.01$ for comparison of the groups. Statistical analysis was done using Student t-test.

erythrocytes to accumulate in circulation, indicated by the significant increase in the proportion of the younger biotin$^{negative}$ erythrocytes. This could indicate either an increased generation of fresh erythrocytes or prolonged life span of younger erythrocytes in blood circulation.

The latter view is again supported by the enhanced reticulocytosis in both cadmium-induced and Paraquat-induced anemia (**Figure 6**). An initial surge of reticulocytes in mice exposed to cadmium and Paraquat was clearly seen. This surge was however lost by the fourth and fifth weeks of cadmium (**Figure 6A**) [17] and Paraquat (**Figure 6B**) [18] exposure, respectively.

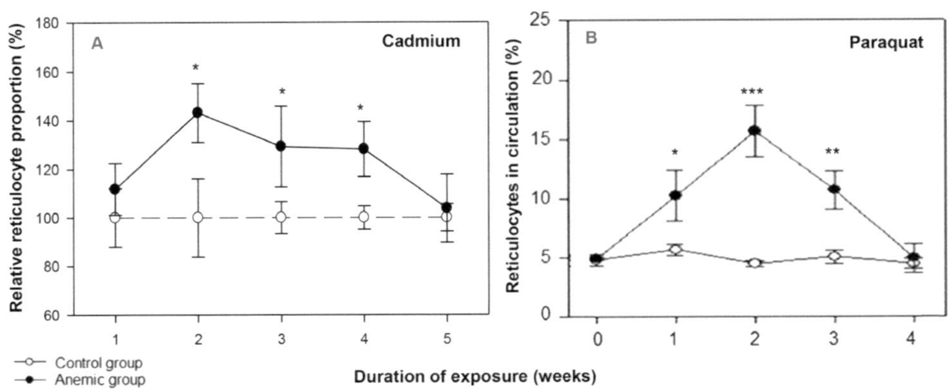


**Figure 6. Circulating reticulocytes in cadmium- and Paraquat-induced anemia**. Mice were rendered anemic by exposure to toxicants like cadmium chloride and Paraquat. Blood was collected at regular interval, and mouse erythrocytes were stained *ex vivo* with anti-mouse CD71-PE to determine the proportion of circulating reticulocytes through flow cytometry. Panel A shows the relative proportions of reticulocytes in cadmium-fed mice. For this, the mean reticulocyte counts in control mice at each time point was taken as 100, and the proportion of reticulocytes in the exposed groups was estimated in relative terms. Panel B shows the reticulocyte proportion in the Paraquat-treated mice. Each point on the graph represents mean ±SEM of observations. n = 10. $^*p < 0.05$, $^{**}p < 0.01$, and $^{***}p < 0.005$ for comparison of the groups. Statistical analysis was done using Student t-test.

## 5.2. Increased susceptibility of young erythrocytes: CNTs and AIHA

Autoimmune hemolytic anemia (AIHA) and anemia induced by exposure to AF-SWCNTs are characterized by a unique turnover profile of circulating erythrocytes, which is radically different from the one observed in Cd- and PQ-induced anemia. There is a significant increase (twofold) in the proportion of older erythrocyte population (biotin$^{high}$, **Figure 7**, panels A and C) along with a concomitant decline in the proportion of young erythrocytes (**Figure 7**, panels B and D). Thus relatively younger erythrocytes in the blood seem to be preferentially eliminated in conditions of AIHA- [20] and CNT-induced anemia [19] either by macrophage-mediated erythrophagocytosis in the reticuloendothelial system of the spleen or by complement-mediated lysis.

In the turnover profile though comparable in both AIHA- and CNT-induced anemia, the two models revealed very different results in terms of the reticulocyte response. The AF-SWCNT treatment resulted in reticulocytosis, showing > twofold increase in the percentage of blood reticulocytes from 2.23 to 5.32% (**Figure 8A**) [19]. Autoimmune anemia on the other hand resulted in severe reticulocytopenia, showing a 16–18% decline in reticulocyte proportion as seen in **Figure 8**, panel B [20].

http://dx.doi.org/10.5772/intechopen.69133

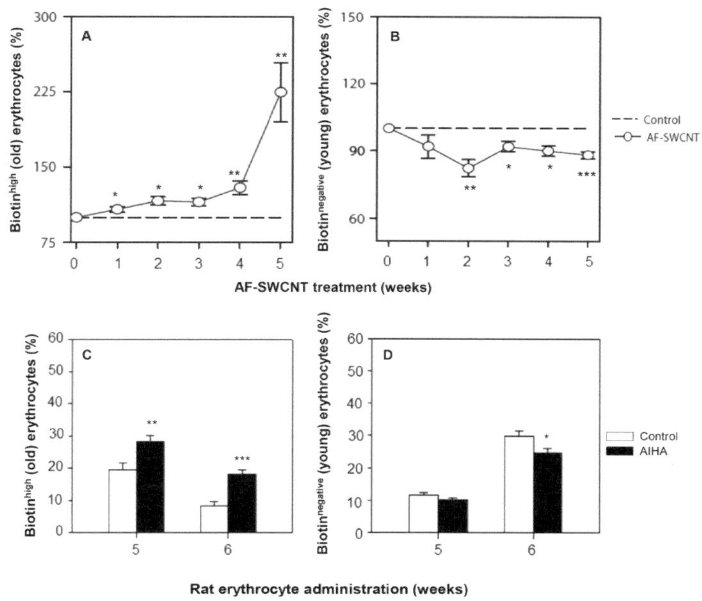


**Figure 7. Erythrocyte turnover in the blood of AIHA mice and mice exposed to AF-SWCNTs.** Mice were rendered anemic by injecting AF-SWCNTs or by inducing AIHA. Mouse erythrocytes were labeled with biotin *in vivo* by the two-step biotinylation procedure (protocol A for CNT-induced anemia; protocol B for AIHA). Erythrocytes were stained *ex vivo* with streptavidin-APC, and proportions of the different age cohorts were determined. Turnover profile of relatively aged biotin$^{high}$ (panels A and C) and young biotin$^{negative}$ (panels B and D) erythrocytes in AF-SWCNT-treated mice (panels A and B) and AIHA mice (panels C and D) has been shown above. The time point for AIHA has been selected on the basis of the induction of anemia (only after the fifth and sixth immunization doses). Each point and each bar on the graph represent mean ±SEM of observations. n = 10. **p* < 0.05, ***p* < 0.01, and ****p* < 0.005 for comparison of the groups. Statistical analysis was done using Student t-test.

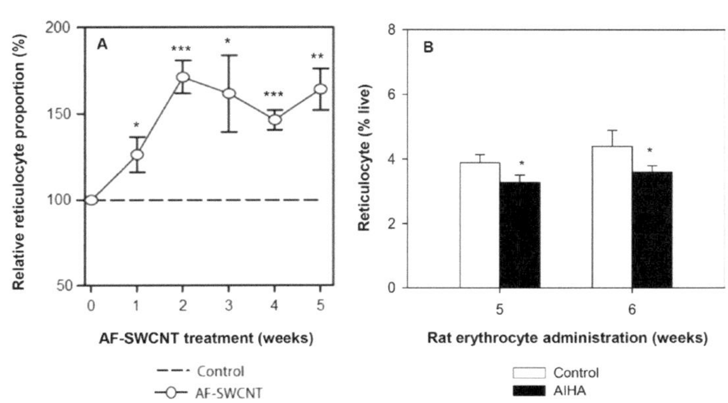


**Figure 8. Circulating reticulocytes in the blood of AIHA mice and mice exposed to AF-SWCNTs.** Mice were rendered anemic by injecting AF-SWCNTs or by inducing AIHA. Blood was collected at regular interval, and mouse erythrocytes were stained *ex vivo* with anti-mouse CD71-PE to determine the proportion of circulating reticulocytes through flow cytometry. Panel A shows the relative proportions of reticulocytes in AF-SWCNT-treated mice. For this, the mean reticulocyte counts in control mice at each time point was taken as 100, and the proportion of reticulocytes in the exposed groups was estimated in relative terms. Panel B shows the reticulocyte proportion in the AIHA mice. The time point for AIHA has been selected on the basis of the induction of anemia (only after the fifth and sixth immunization doses). Each point and each bar on the graph represent mean ±SEM of observations. n = 10. **p* < 0.05, ***p* < 0.01, and ****p* < 0.005 for comparison of the groups. Statistical analysis was done using Student t-test.

## 6. Conclusion

The technique of double *in vivo* biotinylation has been used extensively in our laboratory to unravel the changes associated with erythrocyte aging in circulation. In the present study, the same DIB technique has been used to track the stress-related changes in different age cohorts of erythrocytes and ascertain their susceptibility in different types of anemia. To achieve this goal, we have compared the erythrocyte turnover patterns in four different models of murine anemia, namely anemia induced by (a) toxic heavy metal cadmium (Cd) ions, (b) herbicide Paraquat (PQ), (c) carbon nanotubes (CNTs), and (d) autoantibody in autoimmune hemolytic anemia (AIHA). Interestingly, the study revealed two distinct and contrasting patterns of erythrocyte turnover in murine anemia. This difference could be because of the difference in the way the stress inducers interact with the cell in each of the models. In certain types of anemia, where erythrocytes are exposed to toxicants that directly enter the cells, like in the case of cadmium [73] and Paraquat [74, 75], the stress inducers might interfere with enzyme activities and signaling processes, thereby promoting senescent changes within the cell. Therefore in toxicant stress, as in cadmium-induced anemia and Paraquat-induced anemia, older erythrocytes that are already undergoing senescent changes become more susceptible and are preferentially removed from circulation [17, 18]. On the other hand, in some other cases, where erythrocytes are exposed to agents that directly interact with the cell membrane, as in the case of AIHA- [70, 76] and AF-SWCNT-induced anemia [57], younger erythrocytes in blood circulation are preferentially removed [19, 20]. This biasness could be due to the difference in the membrane composition in the different age cohorts of erythrocytes [77–79]. The fate of the erythrocytes in anemic mice therefore depends on the characteristics and behavior of the stress mediator and therefore may be different in different types of anemia.

## Acknowledgements

The work was funded by three research grants from the Department of Science and Technology (DST), Government of India, to RKS. SC received Senior Research Fellowship from Council of Scientific and Industrial Research (CSIR), New Delhi. Figures used in this manuscript have been compiled from various research publications [11, 12, 14–20].

## Appendices and nomenclatures

| | |
|---|---|
| AF-SWCNT | Acid-functionalized single-walled carbon nanotube |
| AIHA | Autoimmune hemolytic anemia |
| ANOVA | Analysis of variance |
| APC | Allophycocyanin |

| | |
|---|---|
| BXN | Biotin-X-N-hydroxysuccinimide ester |
| CD | Cluster of differentiation |
| Cd | Cadmium |
| $CdCl_2$ | Cadmium chloride |
| CNT | Carbon nanotubes |
| DIB | Double *in vivo* biotinylation |
| FITC | Fluorescein isothiocyanate |
| Ig | Immunoglobulin |
| *i.p.* | Intraperitoneal |
| *i.v.* | Intravenous |
| NHS | N-hydroxysuccinimide |
| PBS | Phosphate-buffered saline |
| PE | Phycoerythrin |
| ppm | Parts per million |
| PQ | Paraquat |
| PS | Phosphatidylserine |
| RES | Reticuloendothelial system |
| ROS | Reactive oxygen species |
| SEM | Standard error of the mean |
| SWCNT | Single-walled carbon nanotube |

## Author details

Sreoshi Chatterjee and Rajiv K. Saxena*

*Address all correspondence to: rajivksaxena@hotmail.com

Faculty of Life Sciences and Biotechnology, South Asian University, New Delhi, India

## References

[1] Goodman JW, Smith LH. Erythrocyte life span in normal mice and in radiation bone marrow chimeras. American Journal of Physiology. 1961;**200**:764-770

[2] Horky J, Vacha J, Znojil V. Comparison of life span of erythrocytes in some inbred strains of mouse using 14C-labelled glycine. Physiologia Bohemoslovenica. 1978;**27**:209-217

[3] Piomelli S, Seaman C. Mechanism of red blood cell aging: Relationship of cell density and cell age. American Journal of Hematology. 1993;**42**:46-52

[4] Clark MR. Senescence of red blood cells: Progress and problems. Physiological Reviews. 1988;**68**:503-554

[5] Morrison M, Jackson CW, Mueller TJ, Huang T, Dockter ME, Walker WS, et al. Does cell density correlate with red cell age? Biomedica Biochimica Acta. 1983;**42**:107-111

[6] Clark MR, Shohet SB. Red cell senescence. Clinics in Haematology. 1985;**14**:223-257

[7] Mueller TJ, Jackson CW, Dockter ME, Morrison M. Membrane skeletal alterations during *in vivo* mouse red cell aging. Increase in the band 4.1a:4.1b ratio. Journal of Clinical Investigation. 1987;**79**:492-499

[8] Suzuki T, Dale GL. Biotinylated erythrocytes: *In vivo* survival and *in vitro* recovery. Blood. 1987;**70**:791-795

[9] Suzuki T, Dale GL. Senescent erythrocytes: Isolation of *in vivo* aged cells and their biochemical characteristics. Proceedings of the National Academy of Sciences of the United States of America. 1988;**85**:1647-1651

[10] Hoffmann-Fezer G, Mysliwietz J, Mortlbauer W, Zeitler HJ, Eberle E, Honle U, et al. Biotin labeling as an alternative nonradioactive approach determination of red cell survival. Annals of Hematology. 1993;**67**:81-87

[11] Khandelwal S, Saxena RK. Assessment of survival of aging erythrocyte in circulation and attendant changes in size and CD147 expression by a novel two step biotinylation method. Experimental Gerontology. 2006;**41**:855-861

[12] Khandelwal S, Saxena RK. A role of phosphatidylserine externalization in clearance of erythrocytes exposed to stress but not in eliminating aging populations of erythrocyte in mice. Experimental Gerontology. 2008;**43**:764-770

[13] Khandelwal S, Saxena RK. Age-dependent increase in green autofluorescence of blood erythrocytes. Journal of Biosciences. 2007;**32**:1139-1145

[14] Khandelwal S, van Rooijen N, Saxena RK. Reduced expression of CD47 during murine red blood cell (RBC) senescence and its role in RBC clearance from the circulation. Transfusion. 2007;**47**(9):1725-1732

[15] Saxena RK, Khandelwal S. Aging and destruction of blood erythrocytes in mice. Current Science. 2009;**97**(4):500-507

[16] Saxena RK, Bhardwaj N, Sachar S, Puri N, Khandelwal S. A Double *in vivo* biotinylation (DIB) technique for objective assessment of aging and clearance of mouse erythrocytes in blood circulation. Transfusion Medicine and Hemotherapy. 2012;**39**:335-341

[17] Chatterjee S, Saxena RK. Preferential elimination of older erythrocytes in circulation and depressed bone marrow erythropoietic activity to cadmium induced anemia in mice. PLoS One. 2015;**10**(7):e0132697

[18] Bhardwaj N, Saxena RK. Elimination of young erythrocytes from blood circulation and altered erythropoietic patterns during paraquat induced anemic phase in mice. PLoS One. 2014;**9**(6):e99364

[19] Bhardwaj N, Saxena RK. Selective loss of younger erythrocytes from blood circulation and changes in erythropoietic patterns in bone marrow and spleen in mouse anemia induced by poly-dispersed single wall carbon nanotubes. Nanotoxicology. 2015;**9**(8):1032-1040

[20] Chatterjee S, Bhardwaj N, Saxena RK. Identification of stages of erythroid differentiation in bone marrow and erythrocyte subpopulations in blood circulation that are preferentially lost in autoimmune hemolytic anemia in mouse. Plos One. 2016;**11**(11):e0166878

[21] IARC. Cadmium and Cadmium Compounds. IARC Monographs Volume 58. 1993. Available from: http://monographs.iarc.fr/ENG/Monographs/vol58/mono58-7.pdf. [Accessed: 21-20-2017]

[22] WHO. Exposure to Cadmium: A Major Public Health Concern. 2010. Availablefrom: http://www.who.int/ipcs/features/cadmium.pdf?ua=1 [Accessed 2017-02-21]

[23] ATSDR. Toxicological Profile for Cadmium. U.S. Department of Health and Human Services, Public Health Service. 2012. Available from: https://www.atsdr.cdc.gov/toxprofiles/tp5.pdf [Accessed 21-02-2017]

[24] Satarug S, Garrett SH, Sens MA, Sens DA. Cadmium, environmental exposure, and health outcomes. Environmental Health Perspectives. 2010;**118**(2):182-190

[25] Franz E, Römkens P, van Raamsdonk L, van der Fels-Klerx I. A chain modeling approach to estimate the impact of soil cadmium pollution on human dietary exposure. Journal of Food Protection. 2008;**71**(12):2504-2513

[26] Järup L, Berglund M, Elinder CG, Nordberg G, Vahter M. Health effects of cadmium exposure—a review of the literature and a risk estimate. Scandinavian Journal of Work, Environment & Health. 1998;**24**(1):1-51

[27] Satarug S, Moore MR. Adverse health effects of chronic exposure to low-level cadmium in foodstuffs and cigarette smoke. Environmental Health Perspectives. 2004;**112**:1099-1103

[28] Sorahan T, Lister A, Gilthorpe MS, Harrington JM. Mortality of copper cadmium alloy workers with special reference to lung cancer and non-malignant diseases of the respiratory system, 1946-92. Occupational and Environmental Medicine 1995;**52**:804-812

[29] J'arup L, Akesson A. Current status of cadmium as an environmental health problem. Toxicology and Applied Pharmacology. 2009;**238**:201-208

[30] Nawrot TS, Staessen JA, Roels HA, Munters E, Cuypers A, Richart T, et al. Cadmium exposure in the population: From health risks to strategies of prevention. Biometals. 2010;**23**:769-782

[31] Horiguchi H, Teranishi H, Niiya K, Aoshima K, Katoh T, Sakuragawa N, et al. Hypoproduction of erythropoietin contributes to anemia in chronic cadmium intoxication: Clinical study on Itai-itai disease in Japan. Archives of Toxicology. 1994;**68**(10):632-636

[32] Horiguchi H, Aoshima K, Oguma E, Sasaki S, Miyamoto K, Hosoi Y, et al. Latest status of cadmium accumulation and its effects on kidneys, bone, and erythropoiesis in inhabitants of the formerly cadmium-polluted Jinzu River basin in Toyama, Japan after restoration of rice paddies. International Archives of Occupational and Environmental Health. 2010;**83**:953-970

[33] Gluhcheva Y, Ivanov I, Atanasov V, Antonova N, Ivanovad Ju, Mitewa M. Hematological changes in case of chronic cadmium intoxication and monensin detoxication. Relationship with rheological variables. Clinical Hemorheology and Microcirculation. 2011;**49**:417-422

[34] Jacobs RM, Fox MRS, Aldridge MH. Changes in Plasma Proteins Associated with the Anemia Produced by Dietary Cadmium in Japanese quail. Journal of Nutrition. 1969;**99**: 119-128

[35] Pond WG, Walker EF Jr., Kirtland D. Cadmium-induced anemia in growing pigs: Protective effect of oral or parenteral iron. Journal of Animal Science 1973;**36**:1122-1124

[36] Sakata S, Iwami K, Enoki Y, Kohzuki H, Shimizu S, Matsuda M, et al. Effects of cadmium on *in vitro* and *in vivo* erythropoiesis: Erythroid progenitor cells (CFU-E), iron, and erythropoietin in cadmium-induced iron deficiency anemia. Experimental Hematology. 1988;**16**:581-587

[37] Horiguchi H, Oguma E, Kayama F. Cadmium and cisplatin damage erythropoietin-producing proximal renal tubular cells. Archives of Toxicology. 2006;**80**:680-686

[38] Horiguchi H, Oguma E, Kayama F. Cadmium Induces Anemia through Interdependent Progress of Hemolysis, Body Iron Accumulation, and Insufficient Erythropoietin Production in Rats. Toxicological Sciences. 2011;**122**(1):198-210

[39] Bismuth C, Garnier R, Baud FJ, Muszynski J, Keyes C. Paraquat poisoning. An overview of the current status. Drug Safety. 1990;**5**:243-251

[40] Dawson AH, Eddleston M, Senarathna L, Mohamed F, Gawarammana I, Bowe SJ, et al. Acute human lethal toxicity of agricultural pesticides: A prospective cohort study. PLoS Medicine 2010;**7**:e1000357

[41] Eddleston M. Patterns and problems of deliberate self-poisoning in the developing world. QJM 2000;**93**:715-731

[42] Bullivant CM. Accidental poisoning by paraquat: Report of two cases in man. British Medical Journal 1966;**1**:1272-1273

[43] Prasad K, Tarasewicz E, Mathew J, Strickland PA, Buckley B, et al. Toxicokinetics and toxicodynamics of paraquat accumulation in mouse brain. Experimental Neurology. 2009;**215**:358-367

[44] Joenje H, Nieuwint AW, Oostra AB, Arwert F, de Koning H, et al. Cytogenetic toxicity of paraquat and streptonigrin in Fanconi's anemia. Cancer Genetics and Cytogenetics. 1987;**25**:37-45

[45] Prihartono N, Kriebel D, Woskie S, Thetkhathuek A, Sripaung N, et al. Risk of aplastic anemia and pesticide and other chemical exposures. Asia-Pacific Journal of Public Health. 2011;**23**:369-377

[46] Baughman RH, Zakhidov AA, de Heer WA. Carbon nanotubes—the route toward applications. Science. 2002;**297**:787-792

[47] Bianco A, Kostarelos K, Prato M. Applications of carbon nanotubes in drug delivery. Current Opinion in Chemical Biology. 2005;**9**:674-679

[48] Kam NW, O'Connell M, Wisdom JA, Dai H. Carbon nanotubes as multifunctional biological transporters and near-infrared agents for selective cancer cell destruction. Proceedings of the National Academy of Sciences of the United States of America. 2005;**102**:11600-11605

[49] Chithrani BD, Ghazani AA, Chan WC. Determining the size and shape dependence of gold nanoparticle uptake into mammalian cells. Nano Letters. 2006;**6**:662-668

[50] Jiang J, Oberdorster G, Elder A, Gelein R, Mercer P, Biswas P. Does nanoparticle activity depend upon size and crystal phase? Nanotoxicology. 2008;**2**:33-42

[51] Sohaebuddin SK, Thevenot PT, Baker D, Eaton JW, Tang L. Nanomaterial cytotoxicity is composition, size, and cell type dependent. Particle and Fibre Toxicology. 2010;**7**:22-39

[52] Davoren M, Herzog E, Casey A, Cottineau B, Chambers G, Byrne HJ, Lyng FM. *In vitro* toxicity evaluation of single walled carbon nanotubes on human A549 lung cells. Toxicology *In Vitro*. 2007;**21**:438-448

[53] Saxena RK, Williams W, Mcgee JK, Daniels MJ, Boykin E, Gilmour MI. Enhanced *in vitro* and *in vivo* toxicity of poly-dispersed acid-functionalized single-wall carbon nanotubes. Nanotoxicology. 2007;**1**(4):291-300

[54] Kumari M, Sachar S, Saxena RK. Loss of proliferation and antigen presentation activity following internalization of polydispersed carbon nanotubes by primary lung epithelial cells. PLoS One. 2012;**7**:e31890

[55] Lam CW, James JT, McCluskey R, Hunter RL. Pulmonary toxicity of single-wall carbon nanotubes in mice 7 and 90 days after intratracheal instillation. Toxicological Sciences 2004;**77**:126-134

[56] Tong H, McGee JK, Saxena RK, Kodavanti UP, Devlin RB, Gilmour MI. Influence of acid functionalization on the cardiopulmonary toxicity of carbon nanotubes and carbon black particles in mice. Toxicology and Applied Pharmacology. 2009;**239**:224-232

[57] Sachar S, Saxena RK. Cytotoxic effect of poly-dispersed single walled carbon nanotubes on erythrocytes *in vitro* and *in vivo*. PLoS One. 2011;**6**(7):e22032

[58] Alam A, Sachar S, Puri N, Saxena RK. Interactions of polydispersed single-walled carbon nanotubes with T cells resulting in downregulation of allogeneic CTL responses *in vitro* and *in vivo*. Nanotoxicology. 2013;**7**:1351-1360

[59] Sokol RJ, Hewitt S. Autoimmune hemolysis: A critical review. Critical Reviews in Oncology/Hematology. 1985;**4**:125-154

[60] Sokol RJ, Booker DJ, Stamps R. The pathology of autoimmune haemolytic Anaemia. Journal of Clinical Pathology. 1992;**45**:1047-1052

[61] Hashimoto C. Autoimmune hemolytic anemia. Clinical Reviews in Allergy & Immunology. 1998;**16**(3):285-295

[62] Gehrs BC, Friedberg RC. Autoimmune hemolytic anemia. American Journal of Hematology. 2002;**69**:258-271

[63] Engelfriet CP, Overbeeke MA, von dem Borne AE. Autoimmune hemolytic anemia. Seminars in Hematology. 1992;**29**:3-12

[64] Izui S, Berney T, Shibata T, Fulpius T, Fossati L, Merino R. Molecular and cellular basis for pathogenicity of autoantibodies. Tohoku Journal of Experimental Medicine 1994;**173**: 15-30

[65] Jefferies LC. Transfusion therapy in autoimmune hemolytic anemia. Hematology/ Oncology Clinics of North America 1994;**8**:1087-1104

[66] Playfair JHL, Marshall-Clarke S. Induction of red cell autoantibodies in normal mice. Nature: New Biology. 1973;**243**:213-214

[67] Weigle WO. Recent observations and concepts in immunological unresponsiveness and autoimmunity. Clinical and Experimental Immunology. 1971;**9**:437-447

[68] Cox KO, Keast D. Erythrocyte autoantibodies induced in mice immunized with rat erythrocytes. Immunology. 1973;**25**:531-539

[69] Naysmith JD, Ortega-Pierres MG, Elson CJ. Rat erythrocyte induced anti-erythrocyte autoantibody production and control in normal mice. Immunology Reviews 1981;**55**: 55-87

[70] Barker RN, Casswell KM, Elson CJ. Identification of murine erythrocyte autoantigens and cross-reactive rat antigens. Immunology. 1993;**78**:568-573

[71] Arndt PA, Garratty G. Flow cytometric analysis in red blood cell immunology. Transfusion Medicine and Hemotherapy. 2004;**31**:163-174

[72] Thedsawad A, Taka A, Wanachiwanawin W. Development of flow cytometry for detection and quantitation of red cell bound immunoglobulin G in autoimmune hemolytic anemia with negative direct Coombs test. Asian Pacific Journal of Allergy and Immunology. 2011;**29**:364-367

[73] Nordberg GF, Kjellstrom T, Nordberg G. Kinetics and metabolism. In: Friberg L, Elinder CG, Kjellstrom T, Nordberg GF, editors. Cadmium and health: A toxicological and epidemiological appraisal. Boca Raton: CRC Press; 1986. pp. 103-178

[74] Chen N, Bowles MR, Pond SM. Prevention of paraquat toxicity in suspensions of alveolar type II cells by paraquat-specific antibodies. Human & Experimental Toxicology. 1994;**13**:551-557

[75] Grabie V, Scemama JL, Robertson JB, Seidel ER. Paraquat uptake in the cultured gastrointestinal epithelial cell line, IEC-6. Toxicology and Applied Pharmacology. 1993;**122**:95-100

[76] Barker RN, Shen C-R, Elson CJ. T-cell specificity in murine autoimmune haemolytic anaemia induced by rat red blood cells. Clinical and Experimental Immunology. 2002;**129**:208-213

[77] Bosman GJCGM, Were JM, Willekens FLA, Novotny VMJ. Erythrocyte ageing *in vivo* and *in vitro*: Structural aspects and implications for transfusion. Transfusion Medicine 2008;**18**:335-347

[78] Bosman GJCGM. Survival of red blood cells after transfusion: Processes and consequences. Frontiers in Physiology. 2013;**4**:376

[79] Lutz HU, Bogdanova A. Mechanisms tagging senescent red blood cells for clearance in healthy humans. Frontiers in Physiology. 2013;**4**:387

Chapter 2

# Immunocamouflaged RBC for Alloimmunized Patients

Mark D. Scott, Wendy M. Toyofuku, Xining Yang,

Meera Raj and Ning Kang

Additional information is available at the end of the chapter

http://dx.doi.org/10.5772/intechopen.68647

**Abstract**

While ABO/Rh(D) red blood cells (RBC)-matched transfusions are generally considered as safe, a significant risk of alloimmunization to non-A/B blood group antigens exists; especially in chronically transfused patients. Indeed, alloimmunization to non-A/B antigens can be so severe that RBC transfusion can no longer be safely administered without the risk of a potentially deadly immune haemolytic reaction. Currently, no satisfactory solutions exist either to prevent blood group alloimmunization or to cost-effectively treat patients with severe alloimmunization. To address this problem, we have pioneered the *immunocamouflage* of donor RBC. The immunocamouflaged (stealth) RBC is manufactured by the covalent grafting of biologically safe polymers to RBC membrane proteins. As a result of the grafted polymer, non-A/B blood group antigens are biophysically and immunologically masked. Of particular interest is the immunocamouflage of the Rh(D) antigen which could be used to improve blood inventory and transfusion safety. The polymer-modified RBCs are morphologically normal and, in mice, exhibit normal *in vivo* survival at immunoprotective grafting concentration. In this chapter, we explore both the biophysical and immunological consequences of the grafted polymers, explore the conditions in which they might be appropriately used, and describe the technology necessary to manufacture functional transfusable units of these cells within the clinical setting.

**Keywords:** red blood cell, immunocamouflage, alloimmunization, Rh(D), polymer

## 1. Introduction

The transfusion of red blood cells (RBC) remains the most common, and best tolerated, form of tissue transplantation. Indeed, an estimated 108 million units of whole blood (~49 million litres) are collected annually worldwide for processing and eventual transfusion [1]. In spite of this massive collection effort, the need for blood constantly exceeds availability due to a combination of collection, manufacturing, storage and, most important clinically, biological (i.e., immunological) issues. The biological challenges facing successful RBC transfusions are vastly underappreciated, largely because of the long history and ubiquity of blood transfusions in modern medicine. Indeed, the RBC is an immunological complex cell with 35 major blood group systems that give rise to over 300 unique antigens capable of eliciting an immune response. Moreover, this immunological complexity is further exacerbated by the finding that the non-A/B (often referred to as *minor*) blood group antigens exist with varying frequencies among different ethnic and racial groups [2, 3]. Within the non-A/B antigens, Rh(D) deserves special attention.

Among the non-A/B blood groups, the Rh system, and in particular Rh(D), is considered to be the most immunogenic antigen. Indeed, the Rh(D) antigen is highly immunogenic and when $Rh(D)^+$ blood is transfused into an $Rh(D)^-$ individual, there is a 50% risk for the development of anti-Rh(D) antibodies resulting in very high risk of a haemolytic transfusion upon a second $Rh(D)^+$ transfusion. Consequent to its immunogenicity, Rh(D) is always determined simultaneously with ABO type and constitutes the '±' found alongside the ABO phenotype. Consequent to its immunogenicity, Rh(D) poses a significant challenge to blood operators since Type O $Rh(D)^-$ ($O^-$) blood is the universal donor cell. In Euro-centric populations, 6–7% of the population is $O^-$ making the maintenance of an adequate inventory of this universal donor blood problematic but possible. Indeed, in North America and Europe, virtually all blood service providers experience a chronic shortage of Type $O^-$ blood. However, in other geographic regions, especially Asia, $Rh(D)^-$ individuals are extremely rare. Indeed, in China, only 0.1–0.4% of the population, regardless of ABO type, is $Rh(D)^-$, making the $Rh(D)^-$ individual (especially with the increasing influx of European tourists) an at-risk patient [4]. Thus, within transfusion medicine, Rh(D) remains a significant problem in terms of both supply and its clinical risk.

Despite the immunological complexity of the RBC, simple ABO/Rh(D) matching has been, typically, considered sufficient for most acute transfusion needs. However, even when ABO/Rh(D) are appropriately matched, transfusion reactions still occur as mismatched non-A/B antigens do carry some immunological risks to a patient. While the incidence of clinically noteworthy (i.e., *significant* patient morbidity) transfusion reactions is relatively low (~0.017% of transfused individuals), less severe transfusion reactions (e.g., transient fever, malaise, premature RBC clearance) and alloimmunization are considerably more frequent and increase with the number of transfusions received by an individual [5–9]. Indeed, with approximately 108 million units of whole blood collected worldwide per annum for blood product preparation, the actual numbers of adverse events become quite significant. Of clinical importance, alloimmunization to non-ABO group antigens is significantly exaggerated in individuals (~30%), especially minorities, receiving chronic transfusion therapy as seen in thalassemia and sickle cell anemia. Indeed, alloimmunization to non-ABO blood groups can be so severe that blood transfusion can no longer be safely administered without risk of a potentially deadly immune haemolytic reaction.

Historically, various interventions have been used in an attempt to prevent transfusion reactions arising from alloimmunization. While ABO/Rh(D) typing has been used since the

1940s, the practice of phenotyping some of the more problematic non-A/B/Rh(D) antigens is still uncommon and likely underlies the high frequency of alloimmunization in chronically transfused patients. In studies on β thalassemia, up to 20% of these chronically transfused individuals demonstrate *clinical* evidence (i.e., mild to severe transfusion reactions) of alloimmunization against non-A/B donor blood group antigens [10, 11]. Rates in patients with sickle cell anemia are even higher (>30%) [12]. As a result, many US National Institutes of Health (NIH) funded Sickle Cell Centres now evaluate a blood recipient for high risk (for alloimmunization) blood group antigens and to prophylactically utilize phenotypically matched blood for transfusion in this cohort of patients. However, even antibody screening does not identify patients alloimmunized to less common RBC antigens or, more importantly, prevent primary alloimmunization to non-tested antigens. To date, the only solutions to prevent alloimmunization, or for individuals with very rare blood type, are to store autologous blood (4°C), maintain an inventory of frozen rare blood group units, keep a blood bank registry of potential donors with rare blood types, utilize extensive RBC phenotyping prior to transfusion and/or encourage minority blood donations [7, 12–27]. While all of these steps are prudent and variably effective, situations still arise where an appropriate (or even satisfactory) blood match cannot be made.

## 2. Bioengineering the red blood cell

Currently, no satisfactory solutions exist to prevent or cost-effectively treat blood group alloimmunization or to improve the inventory of $Rh(D)^-$ blood. To address these unmet needs, the covalent grafting of biocompatible polymers to donor RBC has been proposed to *immunocamouflage* the allogeneic RBC. The immunocamouflaged (stealth) RBC is manufactured by the covalent grafting of methoxypoly(ethylene glycol) [mPEG; PEGylation], as well as other polymers (e.g., polyoxazolines, POZ; and hyperbranched polyglycerols, HPG), to membrane proteins on the surface of allogeneic donor RBC (**Figure 1**).

Most commonly, the chemically activated polymers are covalently grafted to proteins at exposed lysine residues. As a result of the grafted polymer, donor blood group antigens are biophysically and immunologically masked while the modified RBC remaining biologically and functionally viable. To date, most studies have focused on mPEG as the polymer of choice due to its superior ability to both sterically and charge camouflage allogeneic RBC and its well-characterized, and safe, pharmacological profile. The basic chemical structure of mPEG is $HO\text{-}(CH_2CH_2O)_n\text{-}CH_2CH_2CH_3$. mPEG is of low toxicity and is US FDA approved for oral, intravenous, subcutaneous and intramuscular administration [29]. The mPEG polyether polymer is neutrally charged, available in an extraordinarily wide range of molecular weights, and is highly soluble in aqueous-based solutions making it very suitable for pharmacological use. In contrast, both the POZ (e.g., PEOZ) and HPG polymers are poorly soluble in aqueous solutions and only confer weak charge camouflage.

A large number of biological and biophysical studies have been done to characterize the effects of polymer grafting on immune recognition and *in vitro* and *in vivo* viability [28, 30–58]. These studies have demonstrated the significant potential of this immunocamouflage technology in

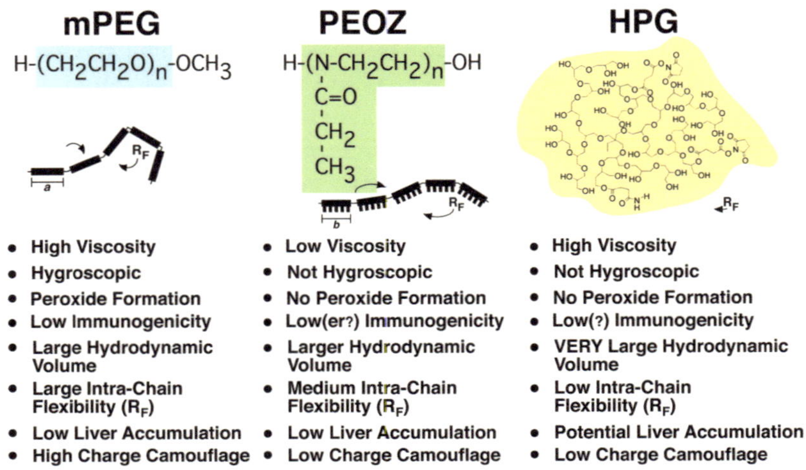


**Figure 1.** Comparison of mPEG, PEOZ and HPG. The repeating structures of mPEG and PEOZ are denoted by the shaded areas while HPG, consisting of repeating polyglycerols, functions more as a mass. The *(a)* and *(b)* notations denote the independent rotational segments of mPEG and PEOZ (respectively) governing intra-chain mobility. The relative intra-chain mobility of the polymers, coupled with polymer size (e.g., 2 versus 20 kDa), underlies the radius of gyration of the grafted polymer. The relative radii of gyrations for mPEG, PEOZ and HPG are indicated by the arrows denoting the Flory radii ($R_F$: root mean square of end-to-end length of the polymer chain) of the polymers. As illustrated, the side-branches of PEOZ decrease intra-chain mobility producing a larger hydrodynamic volume relative to mPEG. Similarly, the highly branched HPG has very limited intra-chain mobility but yields a dense steric 'mushroom'. Modified from Kyluik-Price et al. [28].

transfusion medicine. Example uses include but are not limited to: (1) derivitize RBC to diminish transfusion reactions arising from mismatched blood or alloimmunization; (2) utilization by clinical blood banks to camouflage the Rh(D) antigen to improve blood inventories and utilization; (3) use of mPEG-modified RBC as a 'chain-breaker' (i.e., preventing RBC aggregates arising from abnormal cell-cell interaction) in vascular occlusive diseases such as sickle cell anemia; and (4) prevention of transfusion-associated graft-versus-host disease. Other uses outside of transfusion medicine include the implantation of derivitized cells or cell aggregates (e.g., pancreatic islets) to correct enzyme deficiencies; the induction of tolerance via PEGylated leukocytes; and the prevention of viral infections via antiviral gels.

*Biophysical and biological characterization of the stealth RBC:* The immunocamouflage of cells is a function of the biophysical and biochemical nature of the grafted polymer (**Figure 1**). Biophysically, the grafted polymers confer its immunoprotective effects via both steric hindrance and charge camouflage (**Figure 2**). The efficacy of membrane immunocamouflage is dependent upon both the density (i.e., how much) and depth (i.e., thickness; polymer molecular weight) of the polymer layer. As shown in **Figure 1**, steric hindrance arises from either the rapid mobility arising from intra-molecular flexibility of the polymer (mPEG and PEOZ) and/or polymer density itself (HPG). Perhaps of even more importance is the ability of the polymer to obscure the surface charge (charge camouflage) of the cell. Biophysically, charge camouflage arises from polymer-mediated extension of the shear plane (SP) thereby decreasing the apparent surface charge (**Figure 2A** and **B**). The grafted polymers can give rise to both DIRECT (direct binding to the antigen in question) and INDIRECT (binding to sites other than

http://dx.doi.org/10.5772/intechopen.68647

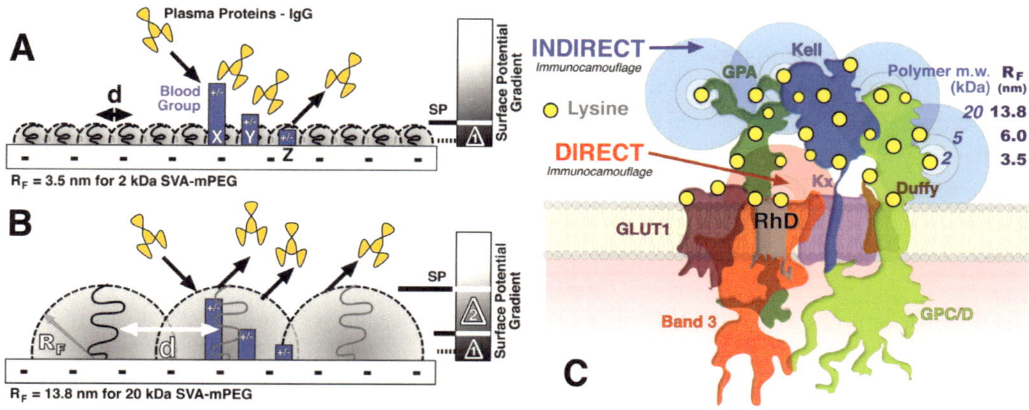


**Figure 2.** Biophysical mechanisms of immunocamouflage. Panels A and B: Prevention of plasma protein (e.g., immunoglobulins) interaction with the cell membrane is due to both steric exclusion (shaded areas induced by the polymers radius of gyration; $R_F$: Flory radii is the root mean square of end-to-end length of the polymer chain) and surface charge camouflage. The effects of both short chain (Panel A) and long chain (Panel B) polymers on the immunocamouflage of surface proteins (X, Y, Z) are schematically shown. The steric effect is maximized when chains are grafted at higher density, that is, with small separation between the chains (d). Importantly, antibody-antigen interaction is, biophysically speaking, charge-mediated. Membrane surface charge camouflage is primarily driven by polymer-mediated extension of the shear plane (SP) toward a region of decreased surface potential (Surface Potential Gradient). In the absence of polymer, the inherent shear plane (SP) of a cell is typically located 1–3 nm above the surface. The extension of SP is proportional to the hydrodynamic thickness of the polymer layer, which in turn is governed by the $R_F$ of the grafted polymer. Thus, 20 kDa polymers (large $R_F$; Panel B) provide improved charge camouflage over 2 kDa polymers (small $R_F$; Panel A). Delta (Δ) is the difference in the surface potential at the shear plane of a particle modified with the short (Δ1) versus the long polymer (Δ2). The membrane proteins X, Y and Z denote blood group antigens extending different distances from the cell surface. Panel C: Not all proteins in the complex topology of the RBC are equally accessible to grafting by the activated polymer, due to either its location in the protein complex or the paucity of lysines (the grafting site of activated mPEG). For example, Rh(D) is deeply buried in the complex while Kell is easily accessible. Thus, *indirect immunocamouflage* maybe more critical than *direct immunocamouflage* (i.e., direct modification of Rh(D) by mPEG) for many blood group antigens. Modified from Refs. [47, 28].

the antigen but conferring indirect camouflage) immunocamouflage of blood group antigens (**Figure 2C**). The importance of indirect immunocamouflage is significant as blood group antigen proteins do not exist in isolation but are most commonly part of complex protein clusters. As shown, the Rh(D) protein is deeply buried within a large protein complex on the surface of the RBC making the direct camouflage of Rh(D) difficult. However, the indirect immunocamouflage of Rh(D) arising from polymers grafted to surrounding proteins (e.g., Kell protein, Band 3) results in the highly efficient immunocamouflage of RhD [28, 52, 55, 59].

Indeed, one of the most promising prospects of RBC immunocamouflage is in both diminishing the risk of Rh(D) alloimmunization and safely increasing blood inventory during emergency situations or in circumstances where Rh(D)$^-$ blood is unavailable. As shown in **Figure 3A**, immune recognition and phagocytosis of anti-D (RhoGAM®; $Rh_o$(D) Immune Globulin (Human) RhoGAM Ultra-Filtered PLUS; Ortho Clinical Diagnostics)-opsonized Rh(D)$^+$ RBC are blocked in a grafting concentration-dependent manner by the grafted mPEG polymer. Importantly, RhoGAM® is a highly purified and concentrated human-derived anti-D IgG antibody that is highly effective at RBC opsonization yielding Monocyte Index (MI) scores in the monocyte-monolayer assay (MMA) in the range of 60–100%. The RhoGAM® antibody is used clinically for the prevention of Rh immunization, including during and after pregnancy and other obstetrical conditions or incompatible transfusion of Rh-positive blood. However, RhoGAM® does not fully reflect the biological/clinical heterogeneity of anti-D alloantibodies arising in alloimmunized individuals. To assess the potential utility of mPEG-RBC in alloimmunized individuals, human-sourced anti-D alloantibodies ($N = 8$) were assessed using the MMA. Of note, the naturally occurring heterogeneity of anti-D responses is demonstrated by the wide range in MI values when used to opsonize Rh(D)$^+$ RBC (**Figure 3B**). Indeed, only five of eight of the alloantibodies exhibited MI values of >5% (i.e., potential for acute haemolytic transfusion reaction). However, as predicted by the RhoGAM findings, grafting of the 20 kDa polymer (2 mM) yielded significant reductions ($p < 0.01$) in the MI values of all samples. Of the five plasma samples with MI values >5%, PEGylation resulted in four having MI values of <5% while the remaining sample had an MI of 5.5 ± 0.9. Moreover, the anti-phagocytic effect of polymer-mediated immunocamouflage of Rh(D)$^+$ RBC was observed regardless of the IgG subclass of the alloantibody. It is also important to note that the serological score (ranging from W+ to 4+) did not correlate significantly with the MI value [59]. These findings are in line with previous studies that demonstrated that the antiglobulin test does not accurately reflect the amount of IgG bound and is, at best, only a weak predictor of RBC phagocytosis [60–63]. In aggregate, these findings suggest that immunocamouflaged Rh(D)$^+$ RBC could be safely transfused into Rh(D)$^-$ patients in an emergency situation.

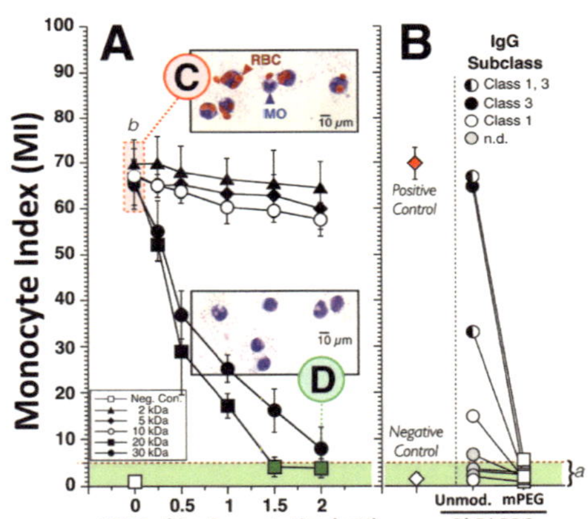


**Figure 3.** Polymer size and grafting concentration governs the efficacy of D immunocamouflage and the inhibition of erythrophagocytosis. Panel A: Effect of polymer size and grafting concentration on MMA phagocytosis of RhoGAM-opsonized Rh(D)$^+$ RBC. As shown, short chain polymers (2–10 kDa) were ineffective at inhibiting erythrophagocytosis. In contrast, membrane modification of Rh(D)$^+$ RBC with both the 20 and 30 kDa mPEG showed a significant ($p < 0.005$ at ≥0.5 mM grafting concentration) dose dependent decrease in phagocytosis. Importantly, the 20 kDa polymer effectively reduced the MI values to ≤5% at grafting concentrations ≥1.5 mM. Interestingly, at equimolar concentration, the 30 kDa polymer was less effective than the 20 kDa polymer. Shown are the mean ± SD of a minimum of three independent experiments. Also shown are representative photomicrographs of an RhoGAM-opsonized Rh(D)$^+$ MMA experiment. Oil-immersion light microscopy of Wright-Giemsa-stained MMA slides. Panel B: Immunocamouflage inhibits erythrophagocytosis of Rh(D)$^+$ RBC opsonized with a diverse array of human anti-D alloantibodies. Similar to the findings with RhoGAM, polymer size is a critical factor in inducing clinically relevant immunocamouflage. Results shown are the mean ± SD for all eight anti-D alloantibodies tested. Also indicated are the IgG subclass of the alloantibodies. The green zone (*a*) indicates MI ≤ 5%, the clinically acceptable range for a non-significant reaction. Panel C: Positive control; multiple monocytes with phagocytized RhoGAM-opsonized Rh(D)$^+$ RBC. Panel D: Shown are the same Rh(D)$^+$ donor RBC as Panel B but modified with mPEG (20 kDa; 2 mM) prior to opsonization. Data derived from Li et al. [59].

Importantly, at immunologically protective grafting concentrations, the grafted polymer does not affect RBC structure or function as evidenced by normal morphology, $O_2$ uptake and delivery, cellular deformability or ion transport [30, 33, 34, 37, 41, 52, 55]. While virtually indistinguishable from unmodified cells in most aspects, one interesting difference was noted between unmodified and mPEG-modified RBC. Consequent to the charge camouflage of the RBC, the cell:cell interactions necessary for Rouleaux formation were abrogated (**Figure 4**). Because the grafted polymer camouflages the charge of the cell necessary for cell:cell interaction, Rouleaux formation is inhibited resulting in attenuation of RBC sedimentation and, physiologically, decreased low-shear viscosity (**Figure 4**). Importantly, the decrease in low-shear viscosity may make the use of stealth RBC highly suitable for patients with diseases characterized by RBC-vaso-occlusive events (e.g., sickle cell). Importantly, RBC PEGylation inhibits both non-antibody (e.g., sickle cell self-aggregation) and antibody-mediated aggregation events and donor mPEG-RBC can serve as an efficient chain-breaker in pro-aggregation states [33].

The grafting of immunologically 'inert' polymers to the membrane of allogeneic RBC effectively camouflages multiple non-ABO antigens from immune recognition. The combined actions of both steric and charge camouflage underlie the ability of the grafted polymer to camouflage allogeneic blood group antigens (immunocamouflage) from the recipient's immune system. These immunocamouflaged (i.e., stealth) RBC may be an effective tool in both preventing and treating alloimmunization in the chronically transfused patient; the transfusion of individual patients with rare blood phenotypes; emergency situation or geographic locations (e.g., China) where $Rh(D)^-$ blood is unavailable. Moreover, immunocamouflaged RBCs are inexpensively and easily manufactured in the clinical setting.

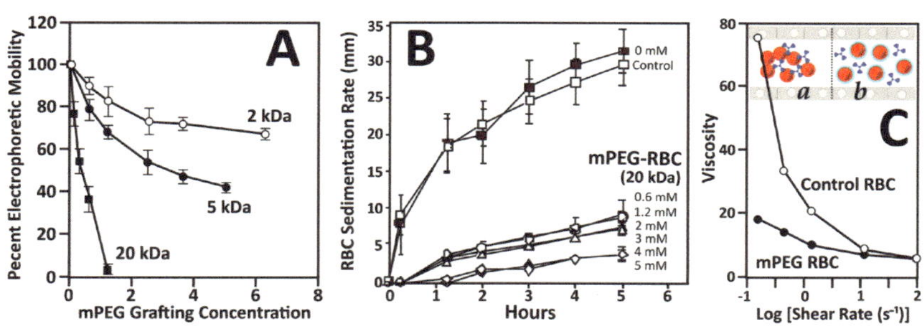


**Figure 4.** Biophysical consequences of RBC PEGylation. Panel A: Charge camouflage of RBC is readily accomplished by polymer grafting and is a function of both grafting concentration and polymer size. As shown, the electrophoretic mobility of the human RBC was completely abrogated by the 20 kDa-activated mPEG at very low grafting concentrations. Mobility of the unmodified human RBC was −1.18±0.12 (μm/s)/(V/cm). Per cent change in mobility was normalized to the mobility of unmodified RBC. Panel B: Polymer grafting prevents cell:cell interaction (Rouleaux formation) via steric and charge camouflage. The loss of Rouleaux formations leads to a dramatically decreased RBC sedimentation rate. Panel C: Low-shear viscosity of the PEG-RBC is significantly reduced in comparison to normal control cells. Control and PEGylated (5 kDa mPEG) RBCs were resuspended to a 40% hematocrit in autologous plasma. Viscosity was measured over a range of shear rates using a Contraves LS30 low-shear viscometer (Contraves AG, Zurich, Switzerland). Data derived from Armstrong et al. [64]. INSERT: PEGylation of RBC alters many characteristics of the RBC. Shown on side *(a)* is the effect of antibody binding to control cells. The RBC agglutinate resulting in a potentially vaso-occlusive event mediated by both antibody binding and enhanced blood viscosity under low-shear conditions. In contrast, as shown on side *(b)*, antibody-mediated aggregation is suppressed in the PEGylated cells, and low-shear viscosity is actually enhanced due to the loss of aggregation and the neutral surface charge of the modified RBC. In addition, the PEGylated cells do not readily interact with the vascular endothelium.

## 3. Manufacturing the 'stealth RBC'

The immunocamouflaged RBC is unlikely to be a *mass-market* product but rather a *boutique blood product for the discriminating customer*. Hence, *on demand* manufacturing of the stealth RBC will be the most likely scenario facing the clinician and blood provider. Fortunately, the manufacturing process of the stealth RBC is rapid and straightforward and requires no specialized equipment on part of the blood provider, hospital or clinic. Moreover, current laboratory tests exist that can, relatively rapidly (~48 h), evaluate the potential clinical utility of the stealth RBC in the at-risk alloimmunized patient. Crucial to the clinical use of the stealth RBC is the manufacturing process. The key tenet of the manufacturing process is the maintenance of a constant polymer:cell ratio in order to achieve a homogenous grafting of the polymers to the individual cells within donor RBC unit (**Figure 5**). If cells are *under-PEGylated*, they retain significant immunogenicity/antigenicity; if cells are *over-PEGylated*, the *in vivo* viability (i.e., circulation time) of the cell is compromised.

To achieve the homogeneity necessary for a clinical mPEG-RBC unit (**Figure 5**), two scalable devices (**Figures 6** and **7**) utilizing micro-mixing chambers (alternatively Y-connectors to induce turbulence and mixing) have been designed, constructed and validated to semi-automate the RBC derivatization process and minimize the risk of contamination. Both approaches can be done aseptically using modifications of existing blood bags and sterile docking devices.

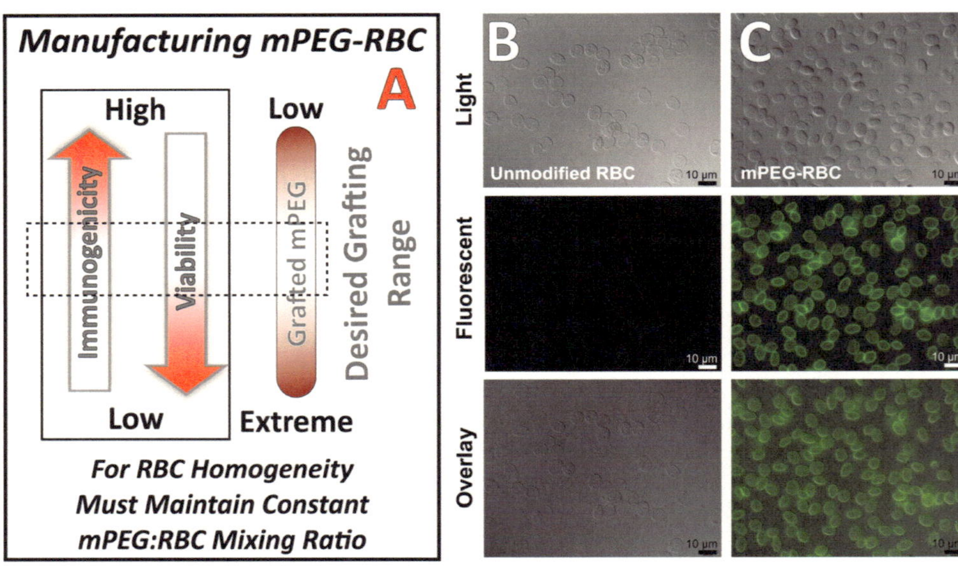


**Figure 5.** Homogeneity of polymer grafting is a critical concern. Extreme grafting levels yield mechanically unstable RBC, while minimally modified RBC retain significant immunologic recognition. To achieve improved grafting homogeneity, 'manufacturing' processes and devices have been developed by our lab. Panels B and C: Using the semi-automated devices described in this chapter, RBCs are uniformly modified by the activated polymer. The uniformity of grafting was documented using an mPEG polymer formulation containing 1% fluorescent 20 kDa mPEG. As shown, the PEGylated RBCs are all fluorescently labeled showing complete derivatization with the semi-automated devices described in this chapter. Modified from Wang et al. [52].

http://dx.doi.org/10.5772/intechopen.68647

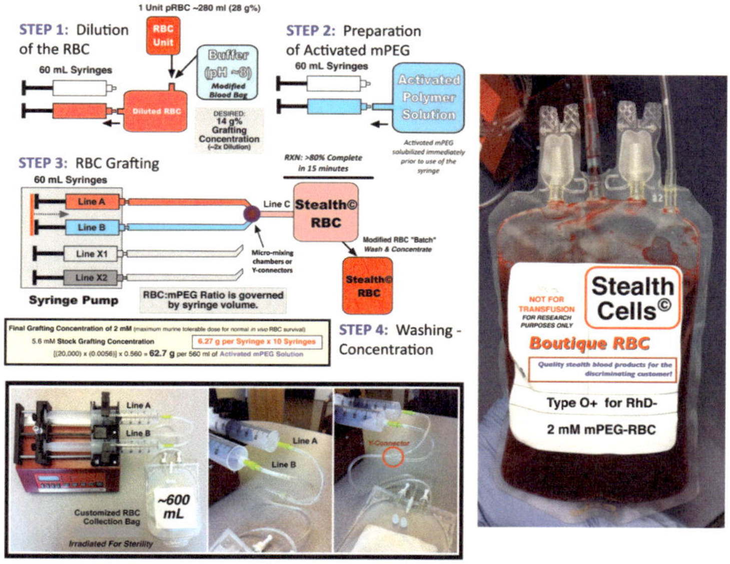


**Figure 6.** Schematic representation for the clinical PEGylation of a single blood unit using the *Syringe Pump Method*. At a minimum, a two-syringe pump is used. Syringe pumps able to handle four or more syringes are commercially available and would speed up the PEGylation process. The syringes can be of either equal or unequal volumes thereby governing the ratio of RBC to activated polymer. The syringe lines lead to the micro-mixing chamber (or Y-connector which will induce turbulence facilitating mixing). The diluted RBC are collected and re-concentrated prior to transfusion. A RBC washing step could be combined with the centrifugation to concentrate the RBC as desired. If desired, a RBC washing step can be combined with the centrifugation step to remove any unreacted polymer though the mPEG is considered safe for injection. Also shown are photographs of the two-syringe pump method and the final stealth RBC blood bag.

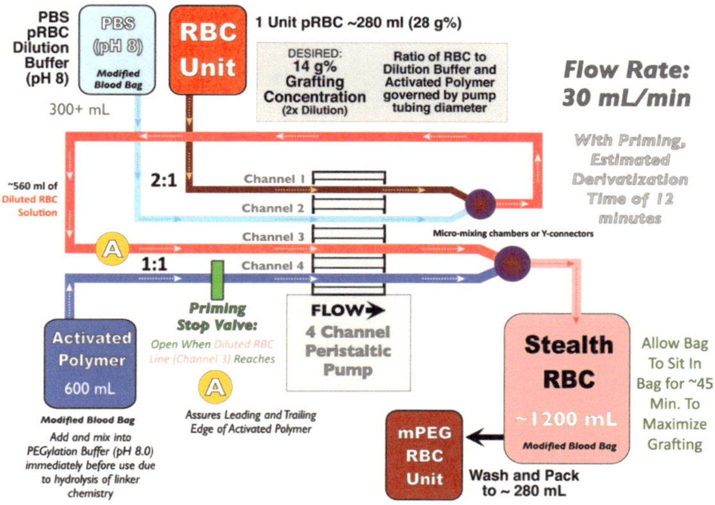


**Figure 7.** Schematic representation for the clinical PEGylation of a single blood unit using the *Four-Channel Peristaltic Pump Method*. Pump tubing used in Channels 1–4 can be of equal or different diameters to govern RBC dilution and the ratio of diluted RBC to activated polymer ratio. A RBC washing step can be combined with a centrifugation process to remove any unreacted polymer though the mPEG is considered safe for injection.

The *Syringe Pump Method* (**Figure 6**) has an advantage in better controlling the hydrolysis rate (i.e., inactivation rate; $t_{1/2}$ of 33 min for succinimidyl valerate-activated methoxypoly(ethylene glycol) [SVAmPEG]) of the activated mPEG as the activated polymer is prepared in smaller batches. The *Peristaltic Pump Method* (**Figure 7**) has the advantage of being a continuous flow device with fewer points of possible disruptions in blood sterility. As demonstrated in **Figure 6**, the described manufacturing devices are capable of producing a transfusable unit of PEGylated RBC.

*RBC manufacturing and product quality control:* Quality assurance of the mPEG-RBC to document the reproducibility and homogeneity of SVAmPEG derivatization can be assessed using a two-phase (PEG-Dextran) partitioning system [37, 41]. The partitioning of PEGylated RBC in this system is governed by the ratio of PEG:Dextran, as well as by the density and size (m.w.; number of ethoxy units) of the grafted mPEG. In this simple assay, mPEG-RBC are added to an immiscible PEG:Dextran solution, rapidly mixed and allowed to separate. As shown, unmodified RBC preferentially partition to the Dextran or interface region while the PEGylated RBC preferentially partition to the PEG-rich phase (**Figure 8**). Importantly, both the automated derivatization and the purification methodologies are highly scalable and can be applied to existing blood bank devices and workflows.

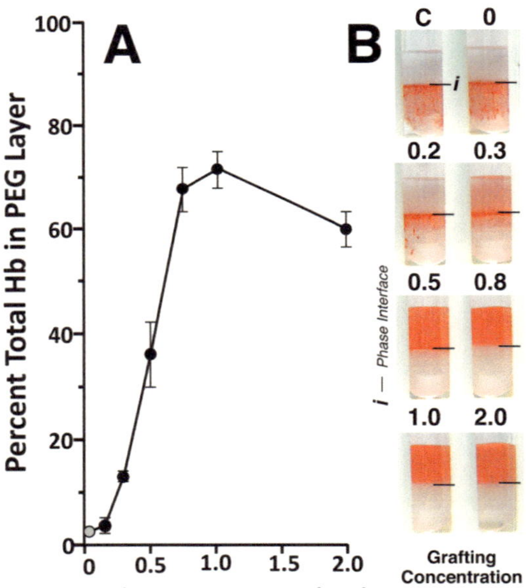


**Figure 8.** Assessing the efficacy of the derivatization reaction via the two-phase PEG-Dextran partitioning system. Panel A: Quantification of phase separation was done via hemoglobin concentration in the PEG layer. Results are expressed as mean ± standard error mean (SEM). Panel B: Representative photos of phase separation of 20 kDa mPEG-RBC over 0–2 mM grafting concentrations. Reflecting increased grafted polymer, the mPEG-RBCs show increased partitioning into the upper PEG layer. Photos were taken 20 min post mixing. Data derived from Bradley and Scott [41] and Kyluik-Price et al. [28].

**The PEGylation Recipe**

**PEGylation Buffer:** While buffer flexibility exists, the chemistry of PEGylation via activated mPEG requires alkaline conditions [28, 30–58]. The formulation of the mPEG-buffer used by our laboratory for the PEGylation of RBC is as follows: 50 mM $K_2HPO_4$, 105 mM NaCl, pH 8.0.

**Activated mPEG:** Following extensive analyses of multiple polymer molecular weights and linker chemistries, 20 kDa succinimidyl valerate-activated methoxypoly(ethylene glycol) [SVAmPEG] has been selected as our primary polymer species. While a wide range of polymer molecular weights (e.g., 2–40 kDa) have been tested, *in vitro* (human and mouse) and *in vivo* (mouse) studies demonstrate that the 20 kDa polymer provides the optimal immunological camouflage of the allogeneic cell while maintaining normal *in vivo* survival. Linker chemistry selection was based on the commercial availability of the polymer, the relatively long half-life of the activated polymer and its excellent *in vitro* and *in vivo* findings. Clinically compliant SVAmPEG can be purchased from *Laysan Bio Inc.* (http://laysanbio.com//; Arab, AL, USA). Because the half-life of the activated polymer upon hydration is short ($t_{1/2}$ of 33 min for SVAmPEG), the polymer should only be solubilized immediately before beginning the grafting event. Specific activated mPEG and buffer volumes for the syringe pump and peristaltic pump method are provided within the method schematics.

## 4. Evaluating the potential clinical utility of the stealth RBC

While multiple studies have demonstrated that RBC immunocamouflage can effectively block immune recognition of multiple blood group antigens, the diversity of alloantibodies produced to a single blood group antigen by humans is staggering. Hence, a crucial step in the clinical use of the stealth RBC should be evaluating the potential efficacy of the stealth cell in the individual patient. While one might assume that standard serological testing techniques would suffice, this is not the case for a variety of reasons. Primary among these reasons, and as shown in **Figure 3C**, is that the laboratory serological score does not correlate significantly with the MI value or the risk of an acute transfusion reaction. Indeed, multiple studies have demonstrated that the antiglobulin test poorly reflects the amount of IgG bound and is, at best, a very weak predictor of RBC phagocytosis [60–63]. This confounding finding is actually by design. Serological testing is 'overly' sensitive in order to detect miniscule amounts of bound antibody to assure the appropriate typing of an individual or to detect the presence of a potentially dangerous alloantibody. Another potential complication is that a large number of commercial testing protocols employ PEG (as either a listed or unlisted ingredient) as a component of the testing reagents. The reagent PEG will cause the mPEG-RBC to segregate as 'PEG likes PEG' (**Figure 8B**). Hence, other predictors of the potential clinical utility of the stealth RBC for an individual patient are needed.

Perhaps the most definitive testing approach for the potential clinical value of the stealth RBC is the monocyte-monolayer assay (MMA). The MMA assesses FcγR-mediated adherence and phagocytosis of alloantibody-opsonized donor RBC by monocytes and has been clinically correlated with *in vivo* transfusion safety (i.e., prevention of acute transfusion reactions) and efficacy (24 h RBC survival) [60–62, 65–68]. The *in vitro* MMA is reliable, reproducible and, within the transfusion medicine community, is considered to be the best assay currently available for the evaluation of FcγR-mediated phagocytosis of antibody-coated human red cells, having more than 20 years of proven validity for the comparison of *in vitro* phagocytosis to *in vivo* clinical relevance.

Schematically, the MMA is described in **Figure 9** (and experimentally demonstrated in **Figure 3**). The MMA examines FcγR-mediated phagocytosis *in vitro* using adherence-purified monocytes isolated from peripheral blood mononuclear cells obtained from normal volunteers. Blood group antigen positive RBCs are incubated with buffer (negative control) or sera or plasma from alloimmunized patients for opsonization, washed and overlaid on the monocyte monolayer. Both donor-obtained and reagent RBC are suitable for use in the MMA. The MMA uses a visual readout whereby the numbers of adherent and phagocytized control and opsonized RBC are enumerated per 100 monocytes (MI). For validation purposes, consistent positive and negative controls should be used, most commonly anti-Rh(D)-opsonized Rh(D)$^+$ (positive control) and Rh(D)$^-$ (negative control) human RBC (see **Figure 3**). The visual inspection is simplified and enhanced by the use of phase contrast microscopy. Using the MMA, MI values of ≤5% indicate that the donor cells can be given without risk of an overt haemolytic reaction. However, it is worth noting that the MMA is most predictive of acute haemolytic transfusion reactions and is less predictive of long-term survival of donor RBC.

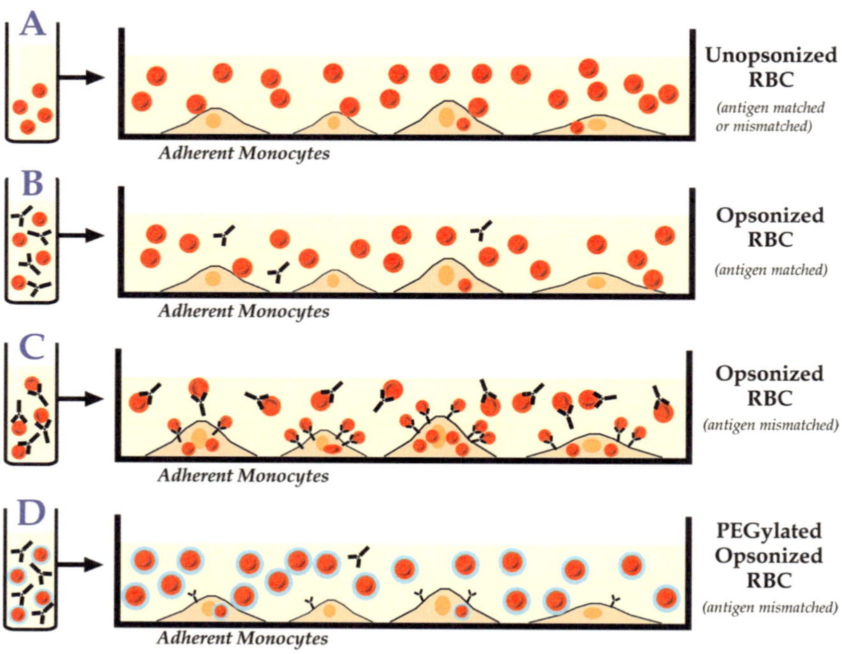


**Figure 9.** Individualized testing of the potential clinical utility of the stealth RBC. Schematic representation of the monocyte-monolayer assay (MMA). (A) Untreated RBC; (B) RBC treated with control (antigen matched) serum or plasma; (C) RBC treated with alloimmunized serum/plasma; and (D) PEGylated RBC treated with alloimmunized serum/plasma. Representative photomicrographs for panels C and D are shown in **Figure** 3.

By using the MMA, the potential efficacy of RBC PEGylation can be done on an individualized basis. The probable success of the stealth RBC transfusion can be further enhanced by serologically selecting (or even better MMA testing) the best possible matches from the donor RBC inventory so as to minimize the risks of additional complications. Once the serological or MMA testing of the donor blood unit has been done, the unit can be PEGylated as described then tested against the individual's alloantibodies via the MMA prior to transfusion into the recipient. However, the identification of the donor unit(s), PEGylation and MMA testing does require 48–96 h lead time. Hence, identification of potential patients should be done as early as possible to assure the availability to source appropriate polymer stock, prepare the PEGylation device and identify and test possible donor units. Concurrent with the evaluation of the potential clinical value of the stealth RBC, the physician/transfusion service must also receive institutional and governmental approval for their use.

## 5. Institutional and governmental approval for patient use

Prior to the actual clinical use of the stealth RBC in a seriously ill patient, compassionate use approval must be obtained from both the hospital Research Ethics Board (REB; or equivalent) and the appropriate governmental agencies (e.g., in Canada, Health Canada). This is likely to be a physician-driven process done in conjunction with the hospital's transfusion service and/or blood provider. Key to these requests is the need to clearly cite the lack of, or very limited availability, of suitable donor RBC. Once institutional approval has been obtained, the hospital REB would likely lead the interaction with the appropriate governmental agency (e.g., Health Canada) regarding an Investigative New Drug (IND) submission. For compassionate use in a single patient who would be likely to die in the absence of a transfusion, a formal IND submission may or may not be necessary. These steps will, obviously, change from country to country.

One question likely to be raised by the REB is whether the proposed mPEG-dosing is safe. The answer to this important question is, at least in part, addressed by recent Phase I–III clinical trials of PEGylated human haemoglobin (PEG-Hb; *Sangart*, San Diego, CA, USA) [69–73]. These clinical trials have infused humans, at the highest dosing schedule, with up to 8.33 ml/kg of PEG-Hb. At this dosing, the typical male volunteers (180 lbs/81.8 kg) received 680 ml of the PEG-Hb solution as a single dose, an infusion of ~25 g of PEG. Importantly, no adverse effects were noted in any of the human volunteers receiving this dose. Furthermore, in animal studies (e.g., rats), PEG-Hb was safely infused at a single adjusted dose exposure of to 46 g of PEG-Hb [74].

## 6. Conclusion

Grafting of immunologically 'inert' polymers to the membrane of allogeneic RBC can effectively camouflage non-ABO antigens from immune recognition. These immunocamouflaged (i.e., stealth) RBCs may be an effective tool in both preventing and treating alloimmunization in the chronically transfused patient; the transfusion of individual patients with rare blood phenotypes; for emergency situation or geographic locations (e.g., China) where

RhD-negative blood is unavailable. Importantly, several characteristics of the immunocamouflaged RBC may also make them highly suitable in patients/diseases characterized by RBC-mediated vaso-occlusive events (e.g., sickle cell) consequent to the polymer-mediated reduction in low-shear viscosity. For the hospital or clinic, the immunocamouflaged RBCs are inexpensively and easily manufactured using commonly available equipment and existing blood bags. Moreover, the potential clinical utility of the stealth RBC can be evaluated for the individual patient using the clinically validated monocyte-monolayer assay in which antigen-mismatched RBCs are PEGylated and then opsonized with the patient's own alloantibody.

## Acknowledgements

The authors would like to thank the past laboratory members whose work as graduate students and postdoctoral researchers have been cited in this chapter: Dr Duncheng Wang, Dr Yevgeniya Le, Dr Dana Kyluik-Price, Dr Li Li, Dr Amanda Bradley, Dr Audrey Chen and Dr Kari Murad. This study was supported by grants from the Canadian Institutes of Health Research (Grant No. 123317; MDS), Canadian Blood Services (MDS) and Health Canada (MDS). The views expressed herein do not necessarily represent the view of the federal government of Canada. We thank the Canada Foundation for Innovation and the Michael Smith Foundation for Health Research for infrastructure funding at the University of British Columbia Centre for Blood Research. The funders had no role in study design, data collection and analysis, decision to publish or preparation of the manuscript.

## Author details

Mark D. Scott*, Wendy M. Toyofuku, Xining Yang, Meera Raj and Ning Kang

*Address all correspondence to: mdscott@mail.ubc.ca

Canadian Blood Services, Centre for Innovation, Pathology and Laboratory Medicine, Centre for Blood Research, University of British Columbia, Vancouver, Canada

## References

[1] Klein HG, Spahn DR, Carson JL. Red blood cell transfusion in clinical practice. Lancet. 2007;**370**:415-426

[2] Reid ME, Lomas-Francis C. The Blood Group Antigen Facts Book. San Diego: Academic Press; 2003

[3] Mourant AE, Kopec AC, Domaniewski-Sobczak K. Blood Groups and Disease. London: Oxford University Press; 1978

[4] Lan JC, Chen Q, Wu DL, Ding H, Pong DB, Zhao T. Genetic polymorphism of RhD-negative associated haplotypes in the Chinese. Journal of Human Genetics. 2000;**45**:2 24-227

[5] NIHCC. Perioperative red cell transfusion. Journal of the American Medical Association. 1988;**260**:2700-2703

[6] Fluit CR, Kunst VA, Drenthe-Schonk AM. Incidence of red cell antibodies after multiple blood transfusion. Transfusion. 1990;**30**:532-535

[7] Vichinsky EP, Earles A, Johnson RA, Hoag MS, Williams A, Lubin B. Alloimmunization in sickle cell anemia and transfusion of racially unmatched blood. New England Journal of Medicine. 1990;**322**:1617-1621

[8] Martin S. Fundamentals of Immunology for Blood Bankers. In: Harmening DM, editor. Modern Blood Banking and Transfusion Practices. Philadelphia, PA. F.A. Davis Company; 1994. p. 43-68.

[9] Moore SB, Taswell HF, Pineda AA, Sonnenberg CL. Delayed hemolytic transfusion reaction. American Society of Clinical Pathologists. 1979;**74**:94-97

[10] Kennedy MS, Julius C. Transfusion Therapy. In: Harmening DM, editor. Philadelphia, PA. F.A. Davis Company; 1994. pp. 316-333.

[11] Economidou J, Constantoulakis M, Augoustaki O, Adinolfi M. Frequency of antibodies to various antigenic determinants in polytransferred patients with homozygous thalassaaemia in Greece. Vox Sanguinis. 1971;**20**:252-258

[12] Luban NL. Variability in rates of alloimmunization in different groups of children with sickle cell disease: Effect of ethnic background. American Journal of Pediatric Hematology-Oncology. 1989;**11**:314-319

[13] Valeri CR, Ragno G, Van Houten P, Rose L, Rose M, Egozy Y, Popovsky MA. Automation of the glycerolization of red blood cells with the high-separation bowl in the Haemonetics ACP 215 instrument. Transfusion. 2005;**45**:1621-1627

[14] Valeri CR. Status report on the quality of liquid and frozen red blood cells. Vox Sanguinis. 2002;**83**(Suppl 1):193-196

[15] Rosenblatt MS, Hirsch EF, Valeri CR. Frozen red blood cells in combat casualty care: Clinical and logistical considerations. Military Medicine. 1994;**159**:392-397

[16] Skrabut EM, Crowley JP, Catsimpoolas N, Valeri CR. The effect of cryogenic storage on human erythrocyte membrane proteins as determined by polyacrylamide-gel electrophoresis. Cryobiology. 1976;**13**:395-403

[17] Valeri CR, Runck AH. Viability of glycerolized red blood cells frozen in liquid nitrogen. Transfusion. 1969;**9**:306-313

[18] Valeri CR, Runck AH. Long term frozen storage of human red blood cells: Studies in vivo and in vitro of autologous red blood cells preserved up to six years with high concentrations of glycerol. Transfusion. 1969;**9**:5-14

[19] Valeri CR, Brodine CE. Current methods for processing frozen red cells. Cryobiology. 1968;**5**:129-135

[20] Beattie KM, Shafer AW. Broadening the base of a rare donor program by targeting minority populations. Transfusion. 1986;**26**:401-404

[21] McPherson ME, Anderson AR, Haight AE, Jessup P, Castillejo MI, Hillyer CD, Josephson CD. Transfusion management of sickle cell patients during bone marrow transplantation with matched sibling donor. Transfusion. 2009;**49**:1977-1986

[22] Anstee DJ. Red cell genotyping and the future of pretransfusion testing. Blood. 2009;**114**: 248-256

[23] Osby M, Shulman IA. Phenotype matching of donor red blood cell units for nonalloimmunized sickle cell disease patients: A survey of 1182 North American laboratories. Archives of Pathology & Laboratory Medicine. 2005;**129**:190-193

[24] Castro O, Sandler SG, Houston-Yu P, Rana S. Predicting the effect of transfusing only phenotype-matched RBCs to patients with sickle cell disease: Theoretical and practical implications. Transfusion. 2002;**42**:684-690

[25] Vichinsky EP, Luban NL, Wright E, Olivieri N, Driscoll C, Pegelow CH, Adams RJ. Prospective RBC phenotype matching in a stroke-prevention trial in sickle cell anemia: A multicenter transfusion trial. Transfusion. 2001;**41**:1086-1092

[26] Rosse WF, et al. Transfusion and alloimmunization in sickle cell disease. Blood. 1990;**76**: 1431-1437

[27] Ambruso DR, Githens JH, Alcorn R, Dixon DJ, Brown LJ, Vaugn WM, Hays T. Experience with donors matched for minor blood group antigens in patients with sickle cell anemia who are receiving chronic transfusion therapy. Transfusion. 1987;**27**:94-98

[28] Kyluik-Price DL, Li L, Scott MD. Comparative efficacy of blood cell immunocamouflage by membrane grafting of methoxypoly(ethylene glycol) and polyethyloxazoline. Biomaterials. 2014;**35**:412-422

[29] Fruijtier-Polloth C. Safety assessment on polyethylene glycols (PEGs) and their derivatives as used in cosmetic products. Toxicology. 2005;**214**:1-38

[30] Scott MD, Murad KL, Koumpouras F, Talbot M, Eaton JW. Chemical camouflage of antigenic determinants: Stealth erythrocytes. Proceedings of the National Academy of Sciences of the United States of America. 1997;**94**:7566-7571

[31] Scott MD, Murad KL. Cellular camouflage: Fooling the immune system with polymers. Current Pharmaceutical Design. 1998;**4**:423-438

[32] Murad KL, Gosselin EJ, Eaton JW, Scott MD. Stealth cells: Prevention of major histocompatibility complex class II-mediated T-cell activation by cell surface modification. Blood. 1999;**94**:2135-2141

[33] Murad KL, Mahany KL, Brugnara C, Kuypers FA, Eaton JW, Scott MD. Structural and functional consequences of antigenic modulation of red blood cells with methoxy poly(ethylene glycol). Blood. 1999;**93**:2121-2127

[34] Scott MD, Bradley AJ, Murad KL. Camouflaged blood cells: Low-technology bioengineering for transfusion medicine? Transfusion Medicine Reviews. 2000;**14**:53-63

[35] Bradley AJ, Test ST, Murad KL, Mitsuyoshi J, Scott MD. Interactions of IgM ABO antibodies and complement with methoxy-PEG-modified human RBCs. Transfusion. 2001;**41**: 1225-1233

[36] Chen AM, Scott MD. Current and future applications of immunological attenuation via pegylation of cells and tissue. BioDrugs. 2001;**15**:833-847

[37] Bradley AJ, Murad KL, Regan KL, Scott MD. Biophysical consequences of linker chemistry and polymer size on stealth erythrocytes: Size does matter. Biochimica et Biophysica Acta. 2002;**1561**:147-158

[38] Chen AM, Scott MD. Immunocamouflage: Prevention of transfusion-induced graft-versus-host disease via polymer grafting of donor cells. Journal of Biomedical Materials Research: Part A. 2003;**67**:626-636

[39] Scott MD, Bradley AJ, Murad KL. Stealth erythrocytes: Effects of polymer grafting on biophysical, biological and immunological parameters. Blood Transfusion. 2003;**1**:244-265

[40] Scott MD, Chen AM. Beyond the red cell: Pegylation of other blood cells and tissues. Transfusion Clinique et Biologique. 2004;**11**:40-46

[41] Bradley AJ, Scott MD. Separation and purification of methoxypoly(ethylene glycol) grafted red blood cells via two-phase partitioning. Journal of Chromatography B: Analytical Technologies in the Biomedical and Life Sciences. 2004;**807**:163-168

[42] McCoy LL, Scott MD. Broad spectrum antiviral prophylaxis: Inhibition of viral infection by polymer grafting with methoxypoly(ethylene glycol). In: Torrence PF, editor. Antiviral Drug Discovery for Emerging Diseases and Bioterrorism Threats. Hoboken, NJ: Wiley & Sons; 2005. pp. 379-395

[43] Chen AM, Scott MD. Comparative analysis of polymer and linker chemistries on the efficacy of immunocamouflage of murine leukocytes. Artificial Cells, Blood Substitutes, and Immobilization Biotechnology. 2006;**34**:305-322

[44] Scott MD. Inactivation of prion proteins via covalent grafting with methoxypoly(ethylene glycol). Medical Hypotheses. 2006;**66**:387-393

[45] Bradley AJ, Scott MD. Immune complex binding by immunocamouflaged [poly(ethylene glycol)-grafted] erythrocytes. American Journal of Hematology. 2007;**82**:970-975

[46] Sutton TC, Scott MD. The effect of grafted methoxypoly(ethylene glycol) chain length on the inhibition of respiratory syncytial virus (RSV) infection and proliferation. Biomaterials. 2010;**31**:4223-4230

[47] Le Y, Scott MD. Immunocamouflage: The biophysical basis of immunoprotection by grafted methoxypoly(ethylene glycol) [mpeg]. Acta Biomaterialia. 2010;**6**:2631-2641

[48] Rossi NA, Constantinescu I, Brooks DE, Scott MD, Kizhakkedathu JN. Enhanced cell surface polymer grafting in concentrated and nonreactive aqueous polymer solutions. Journal of the American Chemical Society. 2010;**132**:3423-3430

[49] Rossi NA, Constantinescu I, Kainthan RK, Brooks DE, Scott MD, Kizhakkedathu JN. Red blood cell membrane grafting of multi-functional hyperbranched polyglycerols. Biomaterials. 2010;**31**:4167-4178

[50] Greco CA, Maurer-Spurej E, Scott MD, Kalab M, Nakane N, Ramirez-Arcos SM. PEGylation prevents bacteria-induced platelet activation and biofilm formation in platelet concentrates. Vox Sanguinis. 2011;**100**:336-339

[51] Kyluik DL, Sutton TC, Le Y, Scott MD. Polymer-mediated broad spectrum antiviral prophylaxis: Utility in high risk environments. In: Carpi A, editor. Progress in Molecular and Environmental Bioengineering—From Analysis and Modeling to Technology Applications. Rijeka: Intech; 2011. pp. 167-190. ISBN 978-953-307-268-5

[52] Wang D, Kyluik DL, Murad KL, Toyofuku WM, Scott MD. Polymer-mediated immunocamouflage of red blood cells: Effects of polymer size on antigenic and immunogenic recognition of allogeneic donor blood cells. Science China Life Sciences. 2011;**54**:589-598

[53] Wang D, Toyofuku WM, Chen AM, Scott MD. Induction of immunotolerance via mPEG grafting to allogeneic leukocytes. Biomaterials. 2011;**32**:9494-9503

[54] Chapanian R, Constantinescu I, Brooks DE, Scott MD, Kizhakkedathu JN. In vivo circulation, clearance, and biodistribution of polyglycerol grafted functional red blood cells. Biomaterials. 2012;**33**:3047-3057

[55] Wang D, Toyofuku WM, Scott MD. The potential utility of methoxypoly(ethylene Glycol)-mediated prevention of rhesus blood group antigen RhD recognition in transfusion medicine. Biomaterials. 2012;**33**:3002-3012

[56] Wang D, Toyofuku WM, Kyluik DL, Scott MD. Use of flow cytometry in the *in vitro* and in vivo analysis of tolerance/anergy induction by immunocamouflage. In: Schmid I, editor. Flow Cytometry-Recent Perspectives. Rijeka, Croatia InTech; 2012. pp. 133-150

[57] Le Y, Toyofuku WM, Scott MD. Immunogenicity of murine mPEG-red blood cells and the risk of anti-PEG antibodies in human blood donors. Experimental Hematology. 2017;**47**:36-47

[58] Kyluik-Price DL, Scott MD. Effects of methoxypoly (ethylene glycol) mediated immunocamouflage on leukocyte surface marker detection, cell conjugation, activation and alloproliferation. Biomaterials. 2016;**74**:167-177

[59] Li L, Noumsi GT, Kwok YY, Moulds JM, Scott MD. Inhibition of phagocytic recognition of anti-D opsonized Rh D+ RBC by polymer-mediated immunocamouflage. American Journal of Hematology. 2015;**90**:1165-1170

[60] Branch DR, Gallagher MT, Mison AP, Sy Siok Hian AL, Petz LD. In vitro determination of red cell alloantibody significance using an assay of monocyte-macrophage interaction with sensitized erythrocytes. British Journal of Haematology. 1984;**56**:19-29

[61] Branch DR, Gallahger MT. Correlation of in vivo alloantibody significance or insignificance with an in vitro monocyte-macrophage phagocytosis assay. British Journal of Haematology. 1986;**62**:783-785

[62] Gallagher MT, Branch DR, Mison A, Petz LD. Evaluation of reticuloendothelial function in autoimmune hemolytic anemia using an in vitro assay of monocyte-macrophage interaction with erythrocytes. Experimental Hematology. 1983;**11**:82-89

[63] Noumsi GT, Billingsley KL, Moulds JM. Successful transfusion of antigen positive blood to alloimmunised patients using a monocyte monolayer assay. Transfusion Medicine. 2015;**25**:92-100

[64] Armstrong JK, Meiselman HJ, Fisher TC. Covalent binding of poly(ethylene glycol) (PEG) to the surface of red blood cells inhibits aggregation and reduces low shear blood viscosity. American Journal of Hematology. 1997;**56**:26-28

[65] Rampersad GC et al. Chemical compounds that target thiol-disulfide groups on mononuclear phagocytes inhibit immune mediated phagocytosis of red blood cells. Transfusion. 2005;**45**:384-393

[66] Karamatic Crew V et al. Two MER2-negative individuals with the same novel CD151 mutation and evidence for clinical significance of anti-MER2. Transfusion. 2008;**48**: 1912-1916

[67] Arndt PA, Garratty G. A retrospective analysis of the value of monocyte monolayer assay results for predicting the clinical significance of blood group alloantibodies. Transfusion. 2004;**44**:1273-1281

[68] Nance SJ, Arndt P, Garratty G. Predicting the clinical significance of red cell alloantibodies using a monocyte monolayer assay. Transfusion. 1987;**27**:449-452

[69] Bjorkholm M, Fagrell B, Przybelski R, Winslow N, Young M, Winslow RM. A phase I single blind clinical trial of a new oxygen transport agent (MP4), human hemoglobin modified with maleimide-activated polyethylene glycol. Haematologica. 2005;**90**:505-515

[70] Olofsson C et al. A multicenter clinical study of the safety and activity of maleimide-polyethylene glycol-modified hemoglobin (hemospan) in patients undergoing major orthopedic surgery. Anesthesiology. 2006;**105**:1153-1163

[71] Olofsson C et al. A randomized, single-blind, increasing dose safety trial of an oxygen-carrying plasma expander (hemospan) administered to orthopaedic surgery patients with spinal anaesthesia. Transfusion Medicine. 2008;**18**:28-39

[72] Vandegriff KD, Malavalli A, Mkrtchyan GM, Spann SN, Baker DA, Winslow RM. Sites of modification of hemospan, a poly(ethylene glycol)-modified human hemoglobin for use as an oxygen therapeutic. Bioconjugate Chemistry. 2008;**19**:2163-2170

[73] Vandegriff KD, Winslow RM. Hemospan: Design principles for a new class of oxygen therapeutic. Artificial Organs. 2009;**33**:133-138

[74] Young MA, Lohman J, Malavalli A, Vandegriff KD, Winslow RM. Hemospan improves outcome in a model of perioperative hemodilution and blood loss in the rat: Comparison with hydroxyethyl starch. Journal of Cardiothoracic and Vascular Anesthesia. 2009;**23**: 339-347

# Chapter 3

# Red Blood Cells and Relation to Thrombosis

Anil Tombak

Additional information is available at the end of the chapter

http://dx.doi.org/10.5772/intechopen.69551

**Abstract**

Blood coagulation and thrombin generation are primarily a function of platelets, coagulation factors, and endothelial cells. Red blood cells (RBCs) have generally been viewed as innocent bystanders in the clotting process. However, there has been a steadily growing clinical data revealing the active roles of erythrocytes in hemostasis. RBCs may contribute to thrombosis in several ways. In polycythemia, RBCs increase blood viscosity and marginate platelets toward the endothelium. The increased incidence of thrombosis is also associated with hemolytic anemia, especially with sickle cell disease and paroxysmal nocturnal hemoglobinuria. RBCs express phosphatidylserine and microparticles, supporting thrombin generation. They interact with platelets, endothelial cells, and fibrinogen, and these interactions lead their incorporation into the thrombi. The presence of RBCs in clots suppresses plasmin generation and reduces clot dissolution. Decreasing thrombus RBC content would accelerate thrombus resolution. In conclusion, RBCs are important complements of the complex reactions of clot formation.

**Keywords:** thrombin, red blood cells, blood coagulation, thrombophilia

## 1. Introduction

Generation of thrombin is a dynamic process that begins with endothelial injury. Endothelial cells, factors in coagulation cascade, platelets, antithrombotic control mechanisms, and fibrinolytic enzymes play major role in this hemostatic process. In addition, various mechanical factors, including blood flow and intercellular molecular bridges, are also involved in the regulation of primary thrombus formation [1]. Red blood cells (RBCs) are the most abundant blood cells, compromising 35–45% of the blood volume. Their plasma membrane has a unique discoid shape, which provides biological and mechanical properties to RBCs necessary to perform their functions [2]. While the major function of RBCs is hemoglobin-mediated oxygen transport through the body, they also actively participate in both arterial and venous thrombosis.

## 2. Evidences and mechanisms for erythrocyte participation in thrombus formation

There has been a steadily growing clinical data revealing the active roles of RBCs in hemostasis. First clinical observation about the role of RBCs in coagulation was published in 1910. In this article, Duke noted that thrombocytopenic patients showed an improvement in bleeding times after transfusion, even though their platelet counts remained low [3]. Fifty years later, Hellem et al. reported decrease in bleeding time upon transfusion of washed RBCs in anemic patients with bleeding defects [4]. The causal factor was again assumed to be the erythrocyte. Ho et al. showed the improved bleeding times after RBC transfusions in patients with anemia and thrombocytopenia [5]. Ho et al. also reported the shortening bleeding time in patients with iron deficiency anemia as their hematocrit increases after iron administration [6]. Anemia increases the risk of bleeding, whereas erythrocytosis increases the risk of thrombosis. When the hematocrit reduced, platelets travel closer to center of the vascular lumen and are thus less likely to interact with the subendothelium [7, 8]. Hemoglobin also scavenges nitric oxide (NO) and therefore a reduced hematocrit would be associated with enhanced NO activity and promoting platelet inhibition and vasodilatation [8]. In addition, red blood cells release adenosine diphosphate (ADP) and thromboxane A2 (TXA2) which enhances platelet aggregation [8]. Weiss et al. corrected a platelet adhesion defect present in patients with a platelet storage pool deficiency by RBC transfusion and concluded about the possible role of ADP [9].

In contrast to patients with low hematocrits, abnormally high RBC counts as in polycythemia vera patients predispose to thrombotic disease [10, 11]. An increase in hematocrit is also associated with cerebral infarction and internal carotid atherosclerosis [12, 13]. In addition, diseases which secondarily alter RBC membrane properties can lead to thrombosis; an increase in RBC aggregation has been associated with thrombosis in retinal venous occlusion, leg vein thrombosis, and coronary heart disease [10, 14–16]. In these disorders, thrombus formation was associated with RBC aggregation that blocks microvascular blood flow. An increase in hematocrit leads to an increase in blood viscosity, an increase in RBC aggregation, and/or a decrease in RBC deformability [10, 17]. Increasing hematocrit promotes the transport of platelets and coagulation factors toward the vessel wall, thereby increasing collisions of platelets with the activated endothelium and with themselves (**Figure 1**) [10, 18, 19]. A decrease in RBC deformability may encourage thrombosis by rendering the erythrocyte less capable of squeezing through narrow apertures [10, 17, 20]. In addition, RBCs have been shown to release adenosine triphosphate (ATP) addition to ADP in response to mechanical deformation, as well [21, 22]. Sickle cell disease (SCD) is a well-known hemoglobinopathy in which the deformability of RBCs decreased, thrombin generation and platelet activation increased. Arterial-venous thrombosis can occur during the vaso-occlusive crisis of SCD. RBC membrane proteins can also promote thrombotic episodes and again SCD is a good example for this; microparticles (MPs) are small membrane vesicles that play important roles on coagulation. RBC and platelet-derived MPs can initiate thrombin generation through factor XIIa, presumably via a phosphatidylserine-mediated process (**Figure 1**) [23]. And sickled RBCs not only shed MPs but also there is an abnormal phosphatidylserine (PS) exposure on RBCs as a result of repeated sickling and unsickling processes [24]. An increase in RBC aggregation and abnormal PS exposure on RBCs have been implicated as possible causative factors of thrombotic complications in beta-thalassemia major cases, as well [10, 25–27]. In addition, under conditions of low $pO_2$ and low pH, which can occur in diseases like hemoglobinopathies, again ATP is secreted by RBCs [28].

Activated platelets express PS on their surfaces which localize the coagulation complexes (intrinsic factor tenase and prothrombinase) to the site of vascular injury and have been viewed as the primary surfaces upon which coagulation occurs [2, 29]. However, normally, a subfraction of RBCs (0.5%) also express PS on their surfaces. With an average RBC count of $\sim 4 \times 10^9$ $mL^{-1}$, this corresponds to approximately $2.5 \times 10^7$ $mL^{-1}$of PS-expressing RBCs, which is 20% of the average platelet count [2]. So, even a small proportion of PS-positive RBCs could significantly affect thrombin generation and promote fibrin deposition during venous thrombosis [2, 30, 31]. Kawakami et al. identified RBCs as having the most active membrane surface among blood cells and endothelial cells in catalyzing the coagulation process in their *in vitro* study, as well [32].

Horne MK et al. also explored the effect of RBC on thrombin generation in clotting whole blood [33]. They not only found that thrombin concentrations increased as the hematocrit increased from 10 to 40% but also found that maximal thrombin concentration increased when red cell lysate mixed with intact red cells or with platelet. The latter effect was lost by filtering the lysate. The authors concluded that it was due to MPs derived from RBCs, and the effect of intact red cells and MPs derived from RBCs on thrombin generation is probably due to the presence of exposed PS on their membranes [33].

Thrombosis is a well-known complication of paroxysmal nocturnal hemoglobinuria (PNH) and has been suggested due to several pathophysiological sates: a suppressed fibrinolytic

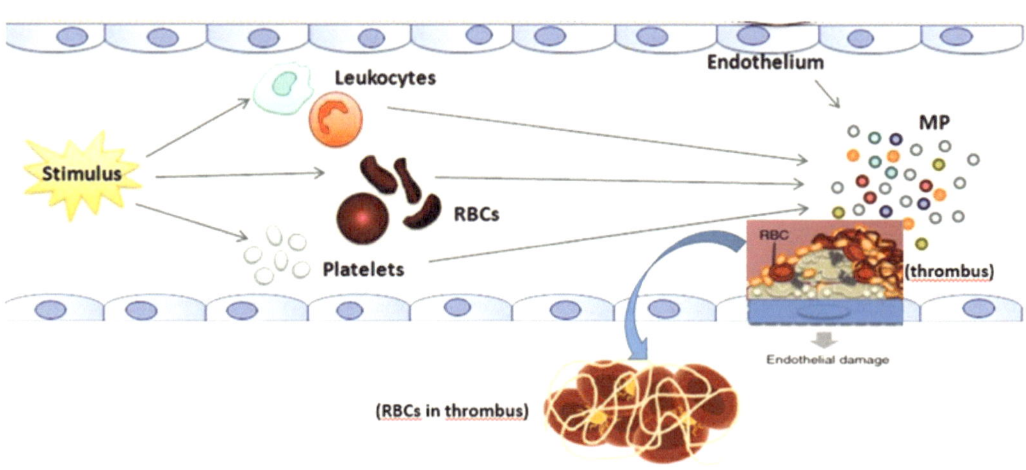


**Figure 1.** In normal conditions, erythrocytes travel in the center of blood flow and platelets travel closer to the endothelial cells. When the hematocrit reduced, platelets travel closer to center of the vascular lumen and are thus less likely to interact with the subendothelium. MPs are small membrane vesicles, which play important roles on coagulation. RBC and platelet-derived MPs can initiate thrombin generation. After formation of the fibrin plaque, RBCs become intertwined within the thrombus to stabilize and strengthen its structure (RBC: red blood cell, MP: microparticle).

system, increased leucocyte-derived tissue factor, complement-mediated damage to platelets and endothelia, and increased platelet derived MPs [34]. Hemolytic attack is often accompanied by thrombosis in PNH and the increased levels of circulating procoagulant MPs derived from hemolyzed RBCs can also contribute thrombophilia by providing the catalytic surface necessary for the assembly of procoagulant, prothrombinase, and tenase enzyme complexes [34]. NO plays an important role in normal platelet functions through the downregulation of platelet aggregation and adhesion. Therefore, NO reduction due to intravascular hemolysis also contributes to thrombogenesis in PNH [34, 35].

Besides all these data about the roles of PS and MPs in thrombogenesis, the erythrocytes do not normally present PS in their outer membrane [10, 36]. For this reason, phospholipid scramblase is required to move the specific aminophospholipids (PS) to an external location. An ATP-requiring mechanism is responsible for this translocation [37] and an increase of the intracellular $Ca^{++}$ concentration in RBC is known to activate the scrambling of membrane phospholipids [37–39]. Phospholipid scrambling plays a stimulatory role in MP generation, as well [40]. Protein kinase C in RBCs mediates the phosphorylation of cytoskeletal proteins and also plays role in $Ca^{++}$ entry into RBCs and subsequent PS exposure on RBC [34, 41, 42].

During clot formation, erythrocytes communicate with platelets as well, and erythrocytes enhance the aggregation of platelets. In the presence of RBCs, greater quantities of free fatty acids and eicosanoid metabolites were generated during platelet activation, rather than in the absence of RBCs [43, 44]. Addition of erythrocytes also enhances platelet degranulation (ADP, serotonin, and beta-thromboglobulin) and aggregation during collagen or thrombin stimulation of platelet-rich plasma [43–48].

RBCs are also incorporated into thrombi via specific interactions during thrombogenesis. RBCs interact with activated endothelial cells (**Figure 2**) and this interaction is demonstrated in a study of arterial thrombosis in which RBCs were the first cells to adhere to a $FeCl_3$-treated intact endothelium, prior to arrival of platelets, and mediate platelet adhesion to the intact endothelial surface [49]. Integrin-mediated interactions between RBCs and leukocytes and platelets may also lead erythrocyte incorporation into thrombi [50]. RBCs bind to platelet $\alpha$IIb$\beta$3 receptor with their intracellular adhesion molecule-4 (ICAM-4) ligand (LW [Landsteiner and Wiener] blood group antigen) and this interaction depends on the platelet activation state [51]. RBC ICAM-4 also interacts with leucocyte $\beta$1 and $\beta$2 integrins [52]. RBCs and fibrinogen also directly interact specifically with each other. Two potential receptors on RBCs have been implicated in fibrinogen-RBC interactions: $\beta$3 or a $\beta$3-like molecule and the integrin-associated protein CD47 [53, 54]. Fibrinogen-mediated transport of factor XIIIa to the clot is necessary for RBC retention in thrombi, as well [55, 56]. Compared to wild-type mice, mice with reduced or delayed factor XIIIa activation produce smaller venous thrombi with reduced RBC content [55]. RBCs affect the structural and mechanical properties of fibrin clots [57]. The interaction of RBCs with fibrin clots (red thrombi) was revealed to be associated with lytic resistance of thrombi due to an increased mechanical strength as compared to clots constituted to plasma only (white thrombi) [58, 59]. In an experimental cerebral ischemia study, it was shown that RBCs within a thrombus transformed from normal discoid shape to form projections which allowed them to interact both with each other and with fibrin fibers. And the authors concluded that through the extension projections, RBCs become intertwined within a thrombus to stabilize and strengthen its structure (**Figure 1**) [57].

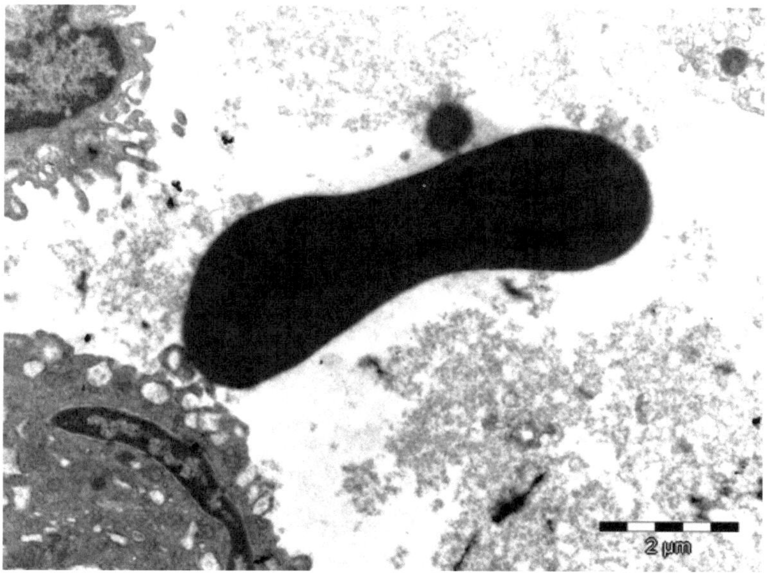


**Figure 2.** Transmission electron microscope of a capillary with a biconcave disk-shaped red blood cell interacting with an endothelial cell (×12,000). By Courtesy of Histology and Embryology Department, Mersin University Medical Faculty.

In summary, RBCs contribute thrombosis by their viscosity effects and by margination of platelets to the vessel wall. However, in addition to these simple viscosity effects of RBC participation in platelet aggregation, RBCs also express PS and MPs, supporting thrombin generation. RBCs interact with platelets, endothelial cells, and fibrinogen, as well and these interactions lead their incorporation into the thrombi. Intertwined RBCs within a thrombus stabilize and strengthens its structure and decrease fibrinolysis. In conclusion, RBCs are important complements of the complex reactions of clot formation.

## Abbreviations

| | |
|---|---|
| RBC | Red blood cell |
| NO | Nitric oxide |
| ADP | Adenosine diphosphate |
| TXA2 | Thromboxane A2 |
| ATP | Adenosine triphosphate |
| SCD | Sickle cell disease |
| MP | Microparticle |
| PNH | Paroxysmal nocturnal hemoglobinuria |
| ICAM-4 | Intracellular adhesion molecule-4 |
| LW | Landsteiner and Wiener |

## Author details

Anil Tombak

Address all correspondence to: aniltombak@mersin.edu.tr

Medical Faculty, Department of Internal Medicine – Hematology, Mersin University, Yenisehir, Mersin, Turkey

## References

[1] Mori D, Yano K, Tsubota K, Ishikawa T, Wada S, Yamaguchi T. Computational study on effect of red blood cells on primary thrombus formation. Thrombosis Research. 2008;**123**:114-121. DOI: 10.1016/j.thromres.2008.03.006

[2] Whelihan MF, Mann KG. The role of the red cell membrane in thrombin generation. Thrombosis Research. 2013;**131**:377-382. DOI: 10.1016/j.thromres.2013.01.023

[3] Duke WW. The relation of blood platelets to hemorrhagic disease. The Journal of the American Medical Association. 1910;**55**:1185-1192

[4] Hellem AJ, Borchgrevink CF, Ames SB. The role of red cells in haemostasis: The relation between haematocrit, bleeding time and platelet adhesiveness. British Journal of Haematology. 1961;**7**:42-50

[5] Ho CH. The hemostatic effect of adequate red cell transfusion in patients with anemia and thrombocytopenia. Transfusion. 1996;**36**:290

[6] Ho CH. Increase of red blood cells can shorten the bleeding time in patients with iron deficiency anemia. Blood. 1998;**91**:1094

[7] Livio M, Gotti E, Marchesi D, Mecca G, Remuzzi G, de Gaetano G. Uraemic bleeding: role of anaemia and beneficial effect of red cell transfusions. Lancet. 1982;**2**:1013-1015.

[8] Kunicki TJ, Nugent DJ. Qualitative Disorders of platelet function. In: Greer JP, Arber DA, Glader B, List AF, Means RT, Paraskevas F, Rodgers GM, editors. Wintrobe's Clinical Hematology. 13th ed. Philadelphia: Lippincott Williams & Wilkins; 2014. p. 1128-1142.

[9] Weiss HJ, Lages B, Hoffman T, Turitto VT. Correction of the platelet adhesion defect in delta-storage pool deficiency at elevated hematocrit-possible role of adenosine diphosphate. Blood. 1996;**87**:4214-4222

[10] Andrews DA, Low PS. Role of red blood cells in thrombosis. Current Opinion in Hematology. 1999;**6**(2):76-82

[11] Schafer AL. Bleeding and thrombosis in the myeloproliferative disorders. Blood. 1984; **64**;1-12

[12] Carallo C, Pujia A, Irace C, Defranceschi MS, Motti C, Gnasso A. Whole blood viscosity and haematocrit are associated with internal carotid atherosclerosis in men. Coronary Artery Disease. 1998;**9**:113-117

[13] Harrison MJG, Pollock S, Kendall BE, Marshall J. Effect of haematocrit on carotid stenosis and cerebral infarction. Lancet. 1981;**2**:114-115

[14] Chabanel A, Glacet-Bernard A, Lelong F, Taccoen A, Coscas G, Samama MM. Increased red blood cell aggregation in retinal vein occlusion. British Journal of Haematology. 1990;**75**:127-131

[15] Chabanel A, Horellou MH, Conard J, Samama MM. Red blood cell aggregability in patients with a history of leg vein thrombosis: Influence of post-thrombotic treatment. British Journal of Haematology. 1994;**88**:174-179

[16] Demiroglu H. The importance of erythrocyte aggregation in blood rheology: Considerations on the pathophysiology of thrombotic disorders. Blood. 1997;**89**:4236

[17] Schmid-Schonbein H, Wells R, Goldstone J. Influence of deformability of human red cell upon blood viscosity. Circulation Research. 1969;**25**:131-143

[18] Goldsmith HL. Red cell motions and wall interactions in tube flow. Federation Proceedings. 1971;**30**:1578-1588

[19] Goldsmith HL, Bell DN, Braovac S, Steinberg A, Mclntosh F. Physical and chemical effects of red cells in the shear-induced aggregation of human platelets. Biophysical Journal. 1995;**69**:1584-1595

[20] Hebbel RP. Beyond hemoglobin polymerization: The red blood cell membrane and sickle cell pathophysiology. Blood. 1991;**77**:214-237

[21] Reimers RC, Sutera SP, Joist SH. Potentiation by red blood cells of shear-induced platelet aggregation: Relative importance of chemical and physical mechanisms. Blood. 1984;**64**:1200-1206

[22] Sprague RS, Ellsworth ML, Stephenson AH, Lonigro AJ. ATP: The red blood cell link to NO and local control of the pulmonary circulation. American Journal of Physiology. 1996;**271**:H2717-H2722

[23] Van Der Meijden PE, Van Schilfgaarde M, Van Oerle R, Renné T, ten Cate H, Spronk HM. Platelet- and erythrocyte-derived microparticles trigger thrombin generation via factor XIIa. J Thromb Haemost. 2012;**10**:1355-1362. DOI: 10.1111/j.1538-7836.2012.04758.x

[24] Whelihan MF, Lim MY, Key NS. Red blood cells and thrombin generation in sickle cell disease. Thrombosis Research. 2014;**133**:S52-S53. DOI: 10.1016/j.thromres.2014.03.021

[25] Chen S, Eldor A, Barshtein G, Zhang S, Goldfarb A, Rachmilewitz E, Yedgar S. Enhanced aggregability of red blood cells of beta-thalassemia major patients. American Journal of Physiology. 1996;**270**:H1951-H1956

[26] Helley D, Eldor A, Girot R, Ducrocq R, Guillin MC, Bezeaud A. Increased procoagulant activity of red blood cells from patients with homozygous sickle cell disease and beta-thalassemia. Thrombosis and Haemostasis. 1996;**76**:322-327

[27] Ruf A, Pick M, Deutsch V, Patscheke H, Goldfarb A, Rachmilewitz EA, Guillin MC, Eldor A. In-vivo platelet activation correlates with red cell anionic phospholipid exposure in patients with beta-thalassaemia major. British Journal of Haematology. 1997;**98**:51-56

[28] Bergfeld GR, Forrester T. Release of ATP from human erythrocytes in response to a brief period of hypoxia and hypercapnia. Cardiovascular Research. 1992;**26**:40-47

[29] Butenas S, Branda RF, van't Veer C, Cawthern KM, Mann KG. Platelets and phospholipids in tissue factor-initiated thrombin generation. Thromb Haemost. 2001;**86**:660-667.

[30] Peyrou V, Lormeau JC, Hérault JP, Gaich C, Pfliegger AM, Herbert JM. Contribution of erythrocytes to thrombin generation in whole blood. Thrombosis and Haemostasis. 1999;**81**;400-406

[31] Whelihan MF, Zachary V, Orfeo T, Mann KG. Prothrombin activation in blood coagulation: The erythrocyte contribution to thrombin generation. Blood. 2012;**120**:3837-3845. DOI: 10.1182/blood-2012-05-427856

[32] Kawakami S, Kaibara M, Kawamoto Y, Yamanaka K. Rheological approach to the analysis of blood coagulation in endothelial cell-coated tubes: Activation of the intrinsic reaction on the erythrocyte surface. Biorheology. 1995;**32**:521-536

[33] Horne MK 3rd, Cullinane AM, Merryman PK, Hoddeson EK. The effect of red blood cells on thrombin generation. British Journal of Haematology. 2006;**133**:403-408

[34] Kozuma Y, Sawahata Y, Takei Y, Chiba S, Ninomiya H. Procoagulant properties of microparticles released from red blood cells in paroxysmal nocturnal haemoglobinuria. British Journal of Haematology. 2011;**152**:631-639. DOI: 10.1111/j.1365-2141.2010.08505.x

[35] Cappellini MD. Coagulation in the pathophysiology of hemolytic anemias. Hematology Am Soc Hematol Educ Program. 2007;**1**:74-78. DOI: 10.1182/asheducation-2007.1.74.

[36] Devaux PF. Static and dynamic lipid asymmetry in cell membranes. Biochemistry. 1991;**30**:1163-1173

[37] Seigneuret M, Devaux PF. ATP-dependent asymmetric distribution of spin-labeled phospholipids in the erythrocyte membrane: Relation to shape changes. Proceedings of the National Academy of Sciences of the United States of America. 1984;**81**:3751-3755

[38] Zhou Q, Zhao J, Stout JG, Luhm RA, Wiedmer T, Sims PJ. Molecular cloning of human plasma membrane phospholipid scramblase. A protein mediating transbilayer movement of plasma membrane phospholipids. Journal of Biological Chemistry. 1997;**272**;18240-18244

[39] Bucki R, Bachelot-Loza C, Zachowski A, Giraud F, Sulpice JC. Calcium induces phospholipid redistribution and microvesicle release in human erythrocyte membranes by independent pathways. Biochemistry. 1998;**37**:15383-15391

[40] Kamp D, Sieberg T, Haest CW. Inhibition and stimulation of phospholipid scrambling activity. Consequences for lipid asymmetry, echinocytosis, and microvesiculation of erythrocytes. Biochemistry. 2001;**40**:9438-9446

[41] Andrews DA, Yang L, Low PS. Phorbol ester stimulates a protein kinase C-mediated agatoxin-TK-sensitive calcium permeability pathway in human red blood cells. Blood. 2002;**100**:3392-3399

[42] de Jong K, Rettig MP, Low PS, Kuypers FA. Protein kinase C activation induces phosphatidylserine exposure on red blood cells. Biochemistry. 2002;**41**:12562-12567

[43] Valles J, Santos MT, Aznar J, Marcus AJ, Martinez-Sales V, Portoles M, Broekman MJ, Safier LB. Erythrocytes metabolically enhance collagen-induced platelet responsiveness via increased thromboxane production, adenosine diphosphate release, and recruitment. Blood. 1991;**78**:154-162

[44] Santos MT, Valles J, Marcus AJ, Safier LB, Broekman MJ, Islam N, Ullman HL, Eiroa AM, Aznar J. Enhancement of platelet reactivity and modulation of eicosanoid production by intact erythrocytes. A new approach to platelet activation and recruitment. Journal of Clinical Investigation. 1991;**87**:571-580

[45] Valles J, Santos MT, Aznar J, Osa A, Lago A, Cosin J, Sanchez E, Broekman MJ, Marcus AJ. Erythrocyte promotion of platelet reactivity decreases the effectiveness of aspirin as an antithrombotic therapeutic modality: The effect of low-dose aspirin is less than optimal in patients with vascular disease due to prothrombotic effects of erythrocytes on platelet reactivity. Circulation. 1998;**97**:350-355

[46] Santos MT, Vallés J, Aznar J, Marcus AJ, Broekman MJ, Safier LB. Prothrombotic effects of erythrocytes on platelet reactivity: Reduction by aspirin. Circulation. 1997;**95**:63-68

[47] Santos MT, Vallés J, Aznar J, Pérez-Requejo JL. Role of red blood cells in the early stages of platelet activation by collagen. Thrombosis and Haemostasis. 1986;**56**:376-381

[48] Pérez-Requejo JL, Aznar J, Santos MT, Vallés J. Early platelet-collagen interactions in whole blood and their modifications by aspirin and dipyridamole evaluated by a new method (BASIC wave). Thrombosis and Haemostasis. 1985;**54**:799-803

[49] Barr JD, Chauhan AK, Schaeffer GV, Hansen JK, Motto DG. Red blood cells mediate the onset of thrombosis in the ferric chloride murine model. Blood. 2013;**121**:3733-3741. DOI: 10.1182/blood-2012-11-468983.

[50] Aleman MM, Walton BL, Byrnes JR, Wolberg AS. Fibrinogen and red blood cells in venous thrombosis. Thrombosis Research. 2014;**133**:S38-S40. DOI: 10.1016/j.thromres.2014.03.017

[51] Hermand P, Gane P, Huet M, Jallu V, Kaplan J, Sonneborn HH, Cartron JP, Bailly P. Red cell ICAM-4 is a novel ligand for platelet-activated alpha IIbbeta 3 integrin. Journal of Biological Chemistry. 2003;**278**:4892-4898

[52] Hermand P, Huet M, Callebaut I, Gane P, Ihanus E, Gahmberg CG, Cartron JP, Bailly P. Binding sites of leukocyte beta 2 integrins (LFA-1, Mac-1) on the human ICAM-4/LW blood group protein. Journal of Biological Chemistry. 2000;**275**:26002-26010

[53] Carvalho FA, Connell S, Miltenberger-Miltenyi G, Pereira SV, Tavares A, Ariëns RA, Santos NC. Atomic force microscopy-based molecular recognition of a fibrinogen receptor on human erythrocytes. ACS Nano. 2010;**4**:4609-4020. DOI: 10.1021/nn1009648

[54] De Oliveira S, Vitorino de Almeida V, Calado A, Rosário HS, Saldanha C. Integrin-associated protein (CD47) is a putative mediator for soluble fibrinogen interaction with human red blood cells membrane. Biochimica et Biophysica Acta. 2010;**1818**:481-490. DOI: 10.1016/j.bbamem.2011.10.028

[55] Aleman MM, Byrnes JR, Wang J-G, Mackman N, Degen JL, Flick MJ, Wolberg AS. Fibrin crosslinking is required for retention of red blood cells in venous thrombi. Blood. 2013;**122**:451

[56] Walton BL, Byrnes JR, Wolberg AS. Fibrinogen, red blood cells, and factor XIII in venous thrombosis. Journal of Thrombosis and Haemostasis. 2015;**13**:S208-S215. DOI: 10.1111/jth.12918

[57] van der Spuy WJ, Pretorius E. Interaction of red blood cells adjacent to and within a thrombus in experimental cerebral ischaemia. Thrombosis Research. 2013;**132**:718-723. DOI: 10.1016/j.thromres.2013.08.024

[58] Gerch KC, Nagaswami C, Weisel JW. Fibrin network structure and clot mechanical properties are altered by incorporation of erythrocytes. Thrombosis and Haemostasis. 2009;**102**:1169-1175. DOI: 10.1160/TH09-03-0199

[59] Wohner N, Sótonyi P, Machovich R, Szabó L, Tenekedjiev K, Silva MM, Longstaff C, Kolev K. Lytic resistance of fibrin containing red blood cells. Arteriosclerosis Thrombosis and Vascular Biology. 2011;**31**:2306-2313. DOI: 10.1161/ATVBAHA.111.229088

Section 2

# Immunomodulatory Properties of Platelets

# Chapter 4

# Platelet and Immunity in Transfusion Medicine

Jinmei Xu, Qunxing An, Wen Yin and Xingbin Hu

Additional information is available at the end of the chapter

http://dx.doi.org/10.5772/intechopen.69135

**Abstract**

Platelets are classically used in the clinic to maintain hemostasis, while recent evidence has shown the important role for platelets in the host inflammatory and immune responses. In fact, platelets in vivo produce different mediators such as cytokines or chemokines, which may be involved in the course of disease treatment, thus platelets transfusion is often an effective therapy in many cases. It is well known that platelets can regulate neutrophils, lymphocytes and other immune cells behavior in immune response, thus directing these immune cells onto the damaged tissues, organs or infected sites. On the other hand, platelets can induce neutrophil extracellular traps release in response to bacterial or viral infection. All the characterized novel profile of platelet, if not all, at least in some situations, should be take into consideration when platelets have to be transfused into patients.

**Keywords:** platelets, inflammation, immunity, transfusion, infection

## 1. Introduction

Platelet is one of the visible components in mammalian blood and is shed from the cytoplasmic cleavage of megakaryocytes in bone marrow. Platelets are small and nucleuses cells with a diameter of 2–3 μm. There are 100–300 × $10^9$/L platelets in human blood circulation system [1, 2]. It was first proposed as platelets by an Italian physician Giulio Bizzozero in 1862 after he found that platelets played an important role in the process of hemostasis after vascular injury [3]. Now, platelets are used to curing dysfunction of blood coagulation, thrombopenia and other diseases in hemostasis. As blood homeostasis greatly depends on platelets (PLT), platelets are routinely transfused and its consumption is enormous in worldwide. There approximately 393375 PLT components were administrated between 2010 and 2012 in the United States America [4], while the transfusion of PLT in China increases dramatically during past years.

To prevent activation *in vitro* before transfusion, platelets are conventionally being maintained at 22 ± 2°C within shaking incubators, and this strategy only can guarantee functional PLT available for 5–7 days. This storage temperature for PLT is a risk because of bacterial contamination. However, bacterial infections after platelet transfusion are rarely reported. There were only 39 transfusion-transmitted bacterial infected cases among the 790854 PLT transfusions [5]. We recorded that the adverse reaction after PLT transfusion was 1% between 2013 and 2015, and bacterial contamination was not observed at all. The main reason undoubtedly is restrictive PLT prepare and administrative procedures. However, the possibility that platelets may have the potency to inhibit bacteria growth is not excluded.

Now, there is gradually recognized that platelets not only participate in hemostasis but also play a role in immune response. Actually, platelets have been reported could help liver macrophages (known as Kuffer cells) to fight against *Bacillus cereus* and methicillin-resistant *Staphylococcus aureus* (MRSA) in mice and platelets were the first cells that contacted with bacteria in liver [6, 7]. Platelets were also identified to contain immune recognition receptors, such as Toll-like receptor 4 (TLR4). Platelets are shedding from megakaryocytes in bone marrow. Each megakaryocyte can produce about 2000 platelets. The content of mRNA is very low in platelet, but it possesses 1/3 transcripts of the whole human genome can encode [8, 9]. There are $\alpha$, $\delta$ and $\lambda$ particles in platelets, and it is well known that microbicidal proteins (PMPs) and antibacterial effect cytokines are contained in the $\alpha$ particles [10]. So it's no strange that platelets may have the functions similar to neutrophilic granulocyte, and behavior more like immune cells [11].

As methicillin-resistant *S. aureus* infection usually results in high mortality, it has been a serious threat to clinical patients and public health. Broad-spectrum antibiotics vancomycin, cefoxitin and tigecycline are used to control MRSA infection, but frequent use of antibiotics is easy to induce drug resistance. Thus the multidrug resistant "super bacterial" was produced. The "super bacterial" is a great threat to human health. Cunningham et al. found that the platelet-rich plasma (PRP) could significantly inhibit the growth of *E. coli* in vitro [12]. In vivo studies using rabbit endocarditis model have shown that platelet-rich plasma could distinctly relieve the early stage endocarditis induced by *S. aureus* [13]. These studies may reveal the antimicrobial effect of platelets, and platelets may be a potential therapeutical agent to retard the regeneration of "super bacterial".

## 2. Platelet is essential to coagulation

The physiological role of platelets is to aggregate, be activated to adhesion and initial the blood clot process on the wound site. Stimulating factors such as hormones, hypoxia, vascular endothelial injury and a variety of proinflammatory cytokines, granules can cause platelet activation. When the injury of blood vessel occurs, the structure of collagen located in vascular endothelium is changed to be easily combined with von Willebrand factor (vWF). Then the vWF/collagen complex is recognized by the glycoprotein Ib $\alpha$ (GPIb$\alpha$), which is expressed on the surface of platelets, to recruit platelets to the injured site. Meanwhile, the collagen receptor glycoprotein VI (GPVI) on the platelets membrane is continuously expressed to make the adhesion of platelets to the injury site more stable. After then, the activation of platelets will happen [14, 15]. Activation of platelets is the key step in the coagulation. This is all depended on the cascade amplification of platelets activation. Once the platelet is activated, its shape changes from discoid to pseudopodium. Meanwhile, the activated platelets release particles to the surrounding environment, thus concentration of adenosine diphosphate (ADP) and thromboxane A2 (TXA2) from the platelets particles get higher in the vicinity, and will combine with the adenonucleotide receptors P2X1 and P2Y12 on the adjacent platelets to induce activation [2, 10, 16]. CD62p (p-selectin) is a common marker for activated platelets, and can be acting as a bridge between platelets and immune cells that contain P-selecting Glycoprotein Ligand-1 (PSGL-1) [17].

Moreover, the number of platelets is negatively related to the severity of the disease. It is gradually clear that platelets will be activated and helpful to recruit immune cells like neutrophils to the infection sites. This illustrated that platelet may be not only simple enough to clot, but it also plays a role in the immune response.

## 3. Platelets express a variety of immune recognition receptors

Platelet cell surface contains a variety of pathogens pattern recognition receptors (pattern recognition receptors, PRRs), such as the Toll-like receptor (TLR) family [18], nucleotide-binding oligomerization domain-like receptor (NLR) family, formyl peptide receptor (FPR) (see in **Figure 1**). These PRRs are helpful to the immune system to resist infection.

TLR is classical of key molecules in human innate immune response to pathogens. Different TLRs could specifically recognize specific pathogens and induce immune cells to secrete different cytokines, resulting in varying degrees of host defense immune response. TLR4 is reported to be existed in both human and mice platelets [19, 20]. TLR4 can effectively recognize Gram-negative bacteria lipopolysaccharide (LPS) and then contribute to acquired immune response. LPS can induce rapid thrombocytopenia, hypotension, and sepsis. In the LPS-induced mouse endotoxemia model, the accumulative platelets in the lung only happened in TLR4 wild-type mice, not in TLR4 deficient animals. LPS could stimulate platelet secretion of dense and granules as indicated by ATP release and P-selectin expression, and thus enhance platelet activation [20, 21]. Platelets express TLR4, CD14, MD2, and MyD88 which are the LPS receptor-signaling complex, and the effect of LPS on platelet activation could be abolished by an anti-TLR4-blocking antibody or TLR4 gene knockout, suggesting that the effect of LPS on platelet aggregation depends on the TLR4 pathway [21]. Recent studies showed platelets TLR4 detected its ligands in blood and induced platelets binding to adherent neutrophils [22]. In addition to TLR4, TLR2 and TLR9 were also detected in platelets.

The NOD2 receptor is a cytoplasmic PRR, mainly recognizing the intracellular antigen and could effectively recognize the Gram-positive bacterial muramyl dipeptide (MDP) to help the body to play immune defense. The NOD2 receptor is mainly expressed in monocytes, macrophages, dendritic cells, intestinal epithelial cells, and paneth cells. But NOD2 receptor in human platelets was identified in recent [23]. The NOD2 receptor is necessary for platelet

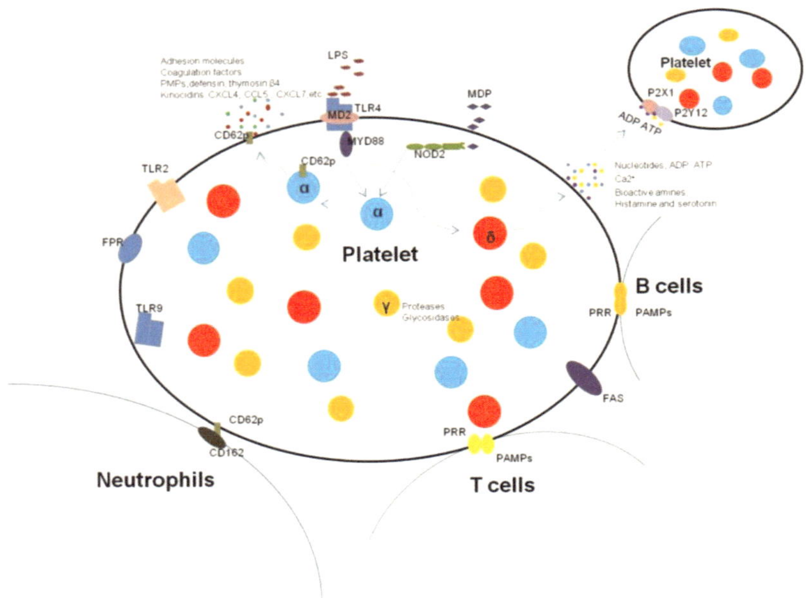


**Figure 1.** The immune receptors and factors in platelets.

aggregation and dense granule release induced by MDP, and the RIP2/MAPK pathway is involved. Different from the NOD2 receptor, there is no NOD1 receptor in the platelets.

In addition to TLR4 and NOD2 receptor, platelet membrane surface also exists formyl peptide receptor (FPR) [24], which plays important role in antimicrobial defense and an apoptosis-related FAS pathway surface receptors exists in platelets too [25]. These immune recognition receptors provide the possibility for the platelet to participate in immune response, which suggests that platelets have the similar function to other immune cells.

## 4. Platelet granules contain special antimicrobial peptide

The platelet granule contains many molecules. Among the three type (α, δ, λ) of granules, nucleotides (such as ADP, ATP, and GTP), bioactive amines (histamine and serotonin) and bioactive ions $Ca^{2+}$ are stored in the δ granules; Enzymes such as proteases and glycosidases are stored in the λ granules; The α granules contain the abundant molecular for hemostasis (for example, adhesion molecules, coagulation factors), the proteins and cytokines for anti-bacterial activity (see in **Figure 1**). The α granules also have molecules such as mitogenic factors and protease inhibitors [26]. The molecules in platelets with antibacterial activity now have been classified as platelet microbicidal proteins (PMPs) and kinocidins [27]. There are kinocidins CXC chemokine ligand 4 (CXCL4; also known as PF-4), CCL5 (also known as RANTES) and CXCL7, and PMPs such as a human defensin, thymosin β4, and fibrinolytic products (FP-A, FP-1) isolated and identified with antibacterial activity [28]. Structural analysis showed that a cationic carboxy-terminal α-helix, which is consistent with peptides that exert direct microbicidal activity. These modular N- and C-terminal regions are an antiparallel β-sheet domain containing the γ-core motif, which is characteristic of all cysteine-stabilized host defense polypeptides in CXCL4 [29]. CCL5 and CXCL4 were detected with high secretion after HIV infection [30]. Human β-defensins displayed classic antimicrobial activity and played a key role in the process of neutrophil extracellular trap formation [31].

Recognition of bacteria by the surface receptor on platelets can activate the platelets effectively and specifically, and induce the release of molecules from platelets granules. Then activation of different types of downstream immune cells indirectly promotes platelets to be involved in immune defense. Studies showed that platelets secrete different type and different doses of molecules when stimulated by different bacteria. When *Escherichia coli* and Salmonella contacted with platelets, the secretion of CCL5 and PDGF were at different levels, while the level of CD62p and CXCL4 were no significant difference. This diversity also exists when peripheral blood mononuclear cells (PBMCs) exposed to the supernatant of platelets contacted with Minnesota Salmonella-induced secrete IL-6, IL-8, and TNFα, while the supernatant of *E. coli* stimulated platelets could not do that [32].

There are many cytokines stored in platelets granules, which the role is not clear yet in hemostasis. For example, transforming growth factor-β (TGF-β), which plays unique and potent immunoregulatory properties, is the most stored in platelets α granules compared to that produced by each leukocyte lineage, including lymphocytes, macrophages, and dendritic cells. The content of TGFβ-1 in platelet is 40-100 times higher than those in other tissues [33, 34]. Increased levels of TGFβ-1 in circulation are usually associated with a wide range of dysfunctional disorders. The level of TGFβ-1 in circulation is always elevated in Marfan syndrome (MFS), coronary heart disease, aortic stenosis and malignancy [35–39]. In contrast, in patients with autoimmune thrombocytopenia, the level of TGFβ-1 in circulation was drastically reduced and increased after treatment [40]. This observation indicates that TGFβ-1 from platelets plays an important role in the immune regulation in diseases. So the role of TGFβ-1 may be helping participate in immune activities, whether TGFβ-1 has an impact on bacteria inhibition is not known yet.

## 5. Antibacterial activity of platelet rich plasma

Platelet-rich plasma (PRP) is used to inhibit bacterium growth in vitro and in vivo [12]. Study of PRP on knee osteoarthritis displayed significant improvement in pain with an effect lasting for up to 6 months [41]. *E. coli* was significantly inhibited in a time-dependent manner when platelets co-cultured with platelet rich plasma (PRP) compared to the platelet poor plasma (PPP). The inhibitory effects increased after co-cultured for 0.5 and 2 h by addition of thrombin to pre-activate platelets in PRP [13]. Studies using rabbit endocarditis model induced by *S. aureus* indicated that platelet-rich plasma could distinctly relieve the early stage endocarditis. In a study of antimicrobial properties of autologous PRP in controlling *S. aureus* with pressure ulcers (PrUs), which is particularly to urine and feces, resulted in increased colonization of wounds, local application of autologous PRP changed the "biological milieu" of the PrUs by its antimicrobial properties, leading to the a reduction of bacterial colonization.

This must be a significant association between PrUs colonization and bacteria present in local environment [42]. An in vitro study of antibacterial properties of PRP on five bacteria (*E. coli, S. aureus, Pseudomonas aeruginosa, Klebsiella pneumoniae* and *Streptococcus faecalis*), indicated that both PRP and PPP inhibited bacterial growth for up to 2 h of incubation. The antimicrobial effect of PRP was significantly higher than that of PPP, and the inoculation concentrations lower or higher, the incubation times longer or shorter are mainly depending on the different bacterial strain. It also indicated that PRP might supply an early protection against bacterial contaminations, because the inhibitory effect is already evident from the first hour of treatment, which may provided the possibility that physiological molecules in PRP might be important in the time interval required for the activation of the innate immune response [12]. As plasma contains antimicrobial peptides and other active substances, the inhibition effect are dependent on platelets or not, is not that clear yet.

## 6. Platelets are involved in inflammation and infection

Clinical studies have shown that bacterial infections, especially sepsis, frequently brought extensive platelet depletion, and the number of platelets is negatively correlated with the severity of the disease [43]. It is known that the sepsis caused by gram-positive bacterium such as *Staphylococcus aureus* often followed by the count reduction of platelets. And infection of gram-negative bacterium *Helicobacter pylori* can induce the immune-thrombopenia [44]. HIV patients are easily detected with drastic platelets number decrease, and this trend is more relevant to the stage of AIDS progress [45]. Similar to HIV infection, infection with Hepatitis C virus (HCV) also lead to the reduction of platelets [46]. It also reported platelets were involved in the fungal infections, such as Aspergillus, Candida, and Cryptococcus [47–50]. As platelets PMPs and kinocidins display sound antibacterial activity, more and more evidence showed that the function of platelets relates to inflammation or infection. Platelets help neutrophils to initial immune defense by secreting a variety of immune associated chemotactic factors, such as β-defensins [31]. Additionally, the link between platelets and neutrophils depends on the combination of CD62p with P-selectin glycoprotein ligand 1 (PSGL1; also known as CD162) molecular on neutrophils. When exposed to the foreign bacterium, platelets are quickly activated and adhere to the wrapped bacterium, while the platelet cell itself occurs intracellular and extracellular membrane rearrangement. Then the CD62p molecular, which rearranges to the platelet membrane surface during the activation of platelets, combines with its ligand PSGL1 to recruit neutrophils to reach the site of infection, and promote the formation of neutrophils extracellular network structure (NET) [51]. After that, it will release antimicrobial substances to kill the bacterium. Platelets can also recruit T cells or B cells (see in **Figure 1**) to reach the site of infection after the bacterial antigens presented by antigen-presenting cells (APCs) such as dendritic cells (DCs) [29, 52–54]. In addition, a recent study reported that there was stem-like megakaryocyte committed progenitors (SL-MkPs) from hematopoietic stem cells (HSCs). SL-MkPs share many features with multipotent HSCs and served as a lineage-restricted emergency pool inflammatory. During homeostasis, SL-MkPs are maintained in a primed but quiescent state, thus contributing little to the megakaryopoiesis in a steady state. Once the inflammation is triggered, SL-MkPs are activated, resulting in megakaryocyte protein production from pre-existing transcripts, then the activated SL-MkPs mature into other megakaryocyte progenitors. This leads to an efficient replenishment of the reduced platelets during inflammatory challenge [55].

## 7. PLT transfusion refractory and immune-related factors

Platelet transfusion is used in cases of very low platelet counts or coagulation dysfunction. The count of platelets is usually performed by a blood cell counter, while thromboela-stogram (TEG) is used for the test of blood clotting function. It has been defined as thrombocytopenia when platelet counts are lower than $150 \times 10^9$/L. Thrombocytopathy appears if a patient has functionally abnormal platelets. Both thrombocytopenia and thrombocytopathy can result in bleeding. Platelet transfusion is suitable for and treatment of thrombocytopenia or platelet dysfunction in patients after or before bleeding, and has become a variety of hematological with chemotherapy and effective supportive therapy for cancer of leukemia patients [56]. But patients in multiple blood transfusion (whole blood, erythrocyte, platelets), pregnancy and organ transplantation, easily produce platelet-related antibodies, resulting in platelet transfusion refractory (PTR). Invalid platelet transfusion refers to the patient in the transfusion of platelets after the platelet count did not effectively improve and the clinical bleeding symptoms did not improve, either. It is generally believed that patients who have received at least two consecutive randomized ABO blood type matched platelets have not achieved a suitable post-transfusion platelet count correction index (CCI) value are considered to be ineffective in platelet transfusion (PTR). At present, the clinical judgment of PTR is mainly the percentage of platelet recovery (PPR or PR%) and CCI [57].

The main causes of PTR can be divided into two categories, non-immune factors, and immune factors. Most PTRs are caused by nonimmunogenic factors, such as the quality of platelet products, hypersplenism, disseminated intravascular coagulation, fever, and antibiotic use. Immune factors include ABO blood type incompatibility, anti-HLA, HPA antibodies, autoantibodies, drug antibodies, allogeneic immune factors. Platelet homologous immunity is equivalent to several times the frequency of erythrocyte antibodies. Antibodies against platelet surface antigens, especially HLA, are the main cause of PTR [57–59]. Platelet-borne antigens can be divided into two major categories: one is the platelet-associated antigen, including HLA class I antigen, as well as ABH, MN, lewis, etc; the other is platelet-specific antigen (HPA), which has a unique type specificity and forms part of the platelet membrane structure. HLA class I antibodies are the most common immune factors that cause PTR, accounting for 80% of all immune factors and 11.7% of all etiologies. PTR caused by HPA antibodies accounts for about 1.7% of all etiologies. Among the HPA types, HPA 1a antigen frequency is > 99.9% in the Chinese population [60, 61], and HPA 2b, 5b, 4b, 3a is not high [62], suggesting that may be the same kind of immune factors lead to the main impact on PTR antigen system.

The current clinical platelet transfusion is a mainly preventive infusion, which become an important means of treatment for thrombocytopenia patients, significantly reducing the mortality of patients with hematological and tumor disorders. However, the pre-procedure platelet transfusion was reported with a high risk of thrombosis and death. In a study of more than 350 hospitalized patients undergoing an invasive procedure, the rate of thrombosis and death increased. Another study of pre-procedure platelet transfusions in a single facility of 376 patients, 19 thrombotic events were appeared up to 5%, this was 21 times greater than the thrombosis rate reported by the Centers of Disease Control and Prevention. So platelets transfusion triggers may need to be reevaluated in non-bleeding patients with available platelet counts [63].

## 8. Summary

Platelets are key factors to maintain hemostasis. Since platelets are involved in infection and inflammation, the immunologic and antimicrobial functions of platelets cannot be ignored when transfused in the clinic. The abundant molecules involved in immune recognition on the platelets surface, such as TLRs, NOD2, CD62p, provide the basis for platelets functional diversity. The functions of bacteria inhibition and performances of anti-infective defense are being more and more recognized. The PMPs and kinocidins from platelets are more potential to be acting as anti-infective agents due to the remarkable immune capability. These natural molecules are safer for the disease control compared to antibiotics, since antibiotics are easily developed into drug-resistance. Moreover, a better understanding of platelets function is helpful to use in diseases therapy. There are also many molecules produced by platelets are unknown, which are deserved to study in the future. In short, the impact of platelets biology on the clinic is profound, and deeply understanding of platelets function will undoubtedly benefit the transfusion medicine.

## Author details

Jinmei Xu, Qunxing An, Wen Yin and Xingbin Hu*

*Address all correspondence to: hxbyqh@fmmu.edu.cn

Department of Transfusion Medicine, Xijing Hospital, China

## References

[1] Yeaman MR. The role of platelets in antimicrobial host defense. Clinical Infectious Diseases: An Official Publication of the Infectious Diseases Society of America. 1997;**25**:951-968; quiz 969-970

[2] Yeaman MR. Platelets in defense against bacterial pathogens. Cellular and Molecular Life Sciences. 2010;**67**:525-544. DOI: 10.1007/s00018-009-0210-4

[3] Semple JW, Italiano JE, Jr, Freedman J. Platelets and the immune continuum. Nature Reviews Immunology. 2011;**11**:264-274. DOI: 10.1038/nri2956nri2956[pii]

[4] Brecher ME, Blajchman MA, Yomtovian R, Ness P, AuBuchon JP. Addressing the risk of bacterial contamination of platelets within the United States: A history to help illuminate the future. Transfusion. 2013;**53**:221-231. DOI: 10.1111/j.1537-2995.2012.03708.x

[5] Harvey AR, Basavaraju SV, Chung KW, Kuehnert MJ. Transfusion-related adverse reactions reported to the National healthcare safety network hemovigilance module, United States, 2010-2012. Transfusion. 2015;**55**:709-718. DOI: 10.1111/trf.12918

[6] Wong CH, Jenne CN, Petri B, Chrobok NL, Kubes P. Nucleation of platelets with blood-borne pathogens on Kupffer cells precedes other innate immunity and contributes to bacterial clearance. Nature Immunology. 2013;**14**:785-792. DOI: 10.1038/ni.2631ni.2631[pii]

[7] Yeaman MR. Platelets: At the nexus of antimicrobial defence. Nature Reviews Microbiology. 2014;**12**:426-437. DOI: 10.1038/nrmicro3269

[8] Alhasan AA, et al. Circular RNA enrichment in platelets is a signature of transcriptome degradation. Blood. 2016;**127**:e1-e11. DOI: 10.1182/blood-2015-06-649434blood-2015-06-649434[pii]

[9] Osman A, et al. Effects of pathogen reduction systems on platelet microRNAs, mRNAs, activation, and function. Platelets. 2015;**26**:154-163. DOI: 10.3109/09537104.2014.898178

[10] Blair P, Flaumenhaft R. Platelet $\alpha$-granules: Basic biology and clinical correlates. Blood Reviews. 2009;**23**:177-189. DOI: 10.1016/j.blre.2009.04.001

[11] Mantovani A, Garlanda C. Platelet-macrophage partnership in innate immunity and inflammation. Nature Immunology. 2013;**14**:768-770. DOI: 10.1038/ni.2666

[12] Mariani E, et al. Platelet-rich plasma affects bacterial growth in vitro. Cytotherapy. 2014;**16**:1294-1304. DOI: 10.1016/j.jcyt.2014.06.003

[13] Aktan Í, Dunkel B, Cunningham FM. Equine platelets inhibit *E. coli* growth and can be activated by bacterial lipopolysaccharide and lipoteichoic acid although superoxide anion production does not occur and platelet activation is not associated with enhanced production by neutrophils. Veterinary Immunology and Immunopathology. 2013;**152**:209-217. DOI: 0.1016/j.vetimm.2012.12.007

[14] Ruggeri ZM. Von Willebrand factor, platelets and endothelial cell interactions. Journal of Thrombosis and Haemostasis. 2003;**1**:1335-1342. DOI: 260 [pii]

[15] Nieswandt B, Varga-Szabo D, Elvers M. Integrins in platelet activation. Journal of Thrombosis and Haemostasis. 2009;**7 Suppl 1**:206-209. DOI: 10.1111/j.1538-7836.2009.03370.xJTH3370[pii]

[16] Yeaman MR. Bacterial-platelet interactions: Virulence meets host defense. Future Microbiology. 2010;**5**:471-506. DOI: 10.2217/fmb.09.112

[17] Stephen J, Emerson B, Fox KA, Dransfield I. The uncoupling of monocyte-platelet interactions from the induction of proinflammatory signaling in monocytes. The Journal of Immunology. 2013;**191**:5677-5683. DOI: 10.4049/jimmunol.1301250jimmunol.1301250[pii]

[18] Aslam R, et al. Platelet Toll-like receptor expression modulates lipopolysaccharide-induced thrombocytopenia and tumor necrosis factor-alpha production in vivo. Blood. 2006;**107**:637-641. DOI: 2005-06-2202 [pii]10.1182/blood-2005-06-2202

[19] Andonegui G, et al. Platelets express functional Toll-like receptor-4. Blood. 2005;**106**:2417-2423. DOI: 2005-03-0916 [pii]10.1182/blood-2005-03-0916

[20] Patrignani P, et al. Reduced thromboxane biosynthesis in carriers of toll-like receptor 4 polymorphisms in vivo. Blood. 2006;**107**:.3572-3574. DOi: 2005-12-4811 [pii]10.1182/blood-2005-12-4811

[21] Zhang G, et al. Lipopolysaccharide stimulates platelet secretion and potentiates platelet aggregation via TLR4/MyD88 and the cGMP-Dependent Protein Kinase Pathway. The Journal of Immunology . 2009;**182**:7997-8004. DOI: 10.4049/jimmunol.0802884

[22] Clark SR, et al. Platelet TLR4 activates neutrophil extracellular traps to ensnare bacteria in septic blood. Nature Medicine. 2007;**13**:463-469. DOI: nm1565 [pii]10.1038/nm1565

[23] Zhang S, et al. Nucleotide-binding oligomerization domain 2 receptor is expressed in platelets and enhances platelet activation and thrombosis. Circulation. 2015;**131**:1160-1170. DOI: 10.1161/CIRCULATIONAHA.114.013743CIRCULATIONAHA.114.013743[pii]

[24] Czapiga M, Gao JL, Kirk A, Lekstrom-Himes J. Human platelets exhibit chemotaxis using functional N-formyl peptide receptors. Experimental Hematology. 2005;**33**:73-84. DOI: S0301-472X(04)00351-0 [pii]10.1016/j.exphem.2004.09.010

[25] Schleicher RI, et al. Platelets induce apoptosis via membrane-bound FasL. Blood 2015;**126**;1483-1493. DOI: 10.1182/blood-2013-12-544445blood-2013-12-544445[pii]

[26] Whiteheart SW. Platelet granules: Surprise packages. Blood. 2011;**118**:1190-1191. DOI: 10.1182/blood-2011-06-359836118/5/1190[pii]

[27] Zhang C, Yang Y. Microparticles are the basic storage units for different proteins in platelet granules. Blood, 2013;**121**:3298. DOI: 10.1182/blood-2012-04-422907

[28] Tang YQ, Yeaman MR, Selsted ME. Antimicrobial peptides from human platelets. Infection and Immunity. 2002;**70**:6524-6533. DOI: 10.1128/iai.70.12.6524-6533.2002

[29] Yeaman MR, Yount NY. Unifying themes in host defence effector polypeptides. Nature Reviews. Microbiology. 2007;**5**:727-740. DOI: nrmicro1744 [pii]10.1038/nrmicro1744

[30] Solomon Tsegaye T, et al. Platelet activation suppresses HIV-1 infection of T cells. Retrovirology. 2013;**10**:48. DOI: 10.1186/1742-4690-10-481742-4690-10-48[pii]

[31] DeLeo FR, et al. Novel Anti-bacterial Activities of β-defensin 1 in Human platelets: Suppression of pathogen growth and signaling of neutrophil extracellular trap formation. PLoS Pathogens. 2011;**7**:e1002355. DOI: 10.1371/journal.ppat.1002355

[32] Berthet J, et al. Human platelets can discriminate between various bacterial LPS isoforms via TLR4 signaling and differential cytokine secretion. Clinical Immunology. 2012;**145**:189-200. DOI: 10.1016/j.clim.2012.09.004S1521-6616(12)00229-X[pii]

[33] Assoian RK, Komoriya A, Meyers CA, Miller DM, Sporn MB. Transforming growth factor-beta in human platelets. Identification of a major storage site, purification, and characterization. The Journal of Biological Chemistry. 1983;**258**:7155-7160

[34] Meyer A, et al. Platelet TGF-beta1 contributions to plasma TGF-beta1, cardiac fibrosis, and systolic dysfunction in a mouse model of pressure overload. Blood. 2012;**119**:1064-1074. DOI: 10.1182/blood-2011-09-377648blood-2011-09-377648[pii]

[35] Fujita S, et al. TGFbeta(1) and sCTLA-4 levels are increased in eltrombopag-exposed patients with ITP. Thrombosis Research. 2012;**130**:415-419. DOI: 10.1016/j.thromres.2012.06.002S0049-3848(12)00273-3[pii]

[36] Rallón NI, et al. Elevated TGF-β1 levels might protect HCV/HIV-coinfected patients from liver fibrosis. European Journal of Clinical Investigation. 2011;**41**:70-76. DOI: 10.1111/j.1365-2362.2010.02381.x

[37] Wang XL, Liu S X, Wilcken DE. Circulating transforming growth factor beta 1 and coronary artery disease. Cardiovascular Research. 1997;**34**:404-410. DOI: S0008636397000333 [pii]

[38] Matt P, et al. Circulating transforming growth factor in Marfan syndrome. Circulation. 2009;**120**:526-532. DOI: 10.1161/circulationaha.108.841981

[39] Lin X, et al. Association between transforming growth factor β1 and atrial fibrillation in essential hypertensive patients. Clinical and Experimental Hypertension. 2014;**37**:82-87. DOI: 10.3109/10641963.2014.913600

[40] Ma L, et al. The cytokines (IFN-gamma, IL-2, IL-4, IL-10, IL-17) and Treg cytokine (TGF-beta1) levels in adults with immune thrombocytopenia. Pharmazie. 2014;**69**:694-697

[41] Patel S, Dhillon MS, Aggarwal S, Marwaha N, Jain A. Treatment with platelet-zich plasma is more effective than placebo for knee osteoarthritis: A prospective, double-blind, randomized trial. The American Journal of Sports Medicine. 2013;**41**:356-364. DOI: 10.1177/0363546512471299036354651247129[pii]

[42] Roop Singh, et al. To evaluate antimicrobial properties of platelet rich plasma and source of colonization in pressure ulcers in spinal injury patients. Hindawi Publishing Corporation. 2015;**2015**:Article ID 749585. 7

[43] Gründler K, et al. Platelet mitochondrial membrane depolarization reflects disease severity in patients with sepsis and correlates with clinical outcome. Critical Care. 2014;**18**:R31. DOI: 10.1186/cc13724

[44] Francois B, et al. Thrombocytopenia in the sepsis syndrome: Role of hemophagocytosis and macrophage colony-stimulating factor. American Journal of Medicine. 199;**103**:114-120. DOI: S0002934397001368 [pii]

[45] Sloand EM, et al. Epidemiology of thrombocytopenia in HIV infection. European Journal of Haematology. 1992;**48**:168-172

[46] Pawlotsky J, et al. Hepatitis C virus infection and autoimmune thrombocytopenic purpura. Journal of Hepatology. 1995;**23**:635-639. DOI: 0168-8278(95)80027-1 [pii]

[47] Speth C, Rambach G, Lass-Flörl C. Platelet immunology in fungal infections. Thrombosis and Haemostasis. 2014;**112**:632-639. DOI: 10.1160/th14-01-0074

[48] Speth C, et al. Aspergillus fumigatus activates thrombocytes by secretion of soluble compounds. The Journal of Infectious Diseases. 2013;**207**:823-833. DOI: 10.1093/infdis/jis743

[49] Carvalho Neiva Tde J, dos Santos JI. Effect of pathogenic yeasts on human platelet aggregation. The Brazilian Journal of Infectious Diseases: An Official Publication of the Brazilian Society of Infectious Diseases. 2003;**7**:370-374

[50] Perkhofer S, et al. Human platelets attenuate aspergillus species via granule-dependent mechanisms. The Journal of Infectious Diseases. 2008;**198**:1243-1246. DOI: 10.1086/591458

[51] Maier M, et al. Platelet factor 4 is highly upregulated in dendritic cells after severe trauma. Molecular Medicine . 2009;**15**:384-391. DOI: 10.2119/molmed.2009.00074

[52] Elzey BD, et al. Platelet-derived CD154 enables T-cell priming and protection against Listeria monocytogenes challenge. Blood. 2008;**111**:3684-3691. DOI: 10.1182/blood-2007-05-091728blood-2007-05-091728[pii]

[53] Elzey BD, Ratliff TL, Sowa JM, Crist SA. Platelet CD40L at the interface of adaptive immunity. Thrombosis Research. 2011;**127**:180-183. DOI: 10.1016/j.thromres.2010.10.011

[54] Wang Z, et al. Essential roles for platelets during neutrophil-dependent or lymphocyte-mediated defense against bacterial pathogens. Blood Coagulation Fibrinolysis. 2016;**27**:667-672. DOI: 10.1097/MBC.0000000000000455

[55] Haas S, et al. Inflammation-induced emergency megakaryopoiesis driven by hematopoietic stem cell-like megakaryocyte progenitors. Cell Stem Cell. 2015;**17**:422-434. DOI: 10.1016/j.stem.2015.07.007

[56] Maxime Berthelot-Richer, et al. Romiplostim efficacy in an acute myeloid leukemia patient with transfusion refractory thrombocytopenia. Transfusion. 2012;**52**:739-741

[57] Jeremy Ryan A, et al. Anti-HLA alloantibodies in surgical patients refractory to platelet transfusion. American Journal of Hematology. 2014;**89**(9):E133-E137

[58] Julie Di Cristofaro, et al. Identification of anti-HPA-1a allo-antibodies using IgG platelet antibody detection and crossmatch system assay with Galileo Echo. Platelets. 2015; **26**(5):421-424

[59] Christiane Gras, et al. HLA-universal platelet transfusions prevent platelet refractoriness in a mouse model. Human Gene Therapy. 2013;**24**:1018-1028.

[60] Guoguang Wu, et al. Platelet immunology in China: research and clinical applications. Transfusion Medicine Reviews. 2017;**31**:118-125

[61] Xia WJ, et al. Establishment of platelet donor registry improves the treatment of platelet transfusion refractorines in Guangzhou region of China. Transfusion Medicine. 2010;**20**:269-274

[62] Sarra Saidi, et al. Polymorphisms of the human platelet alloantigens HPA-1, HPA-2, HPA-3, and HPA-4 in ischemic stroke. American Journal of Hematology. 2008;**83**:570-573

[63] Kerri Waatchter. Annual meeting research trakles non-infectious adverse events. AABB News. 2017;**19**(1)

Section 3

# Transfusion Strategies

Chapter 5

# Red Blood Cell Transfusion and Functional Dose

Deqing Wang and Leiying Zhang

Additional information is available at the end of the chapter

http://dx.doi.org/10.5772/intechopen.68805

**Abstract**

**Objective:** The objective is to study the relationship between cell age and function in the process of the red blood cell (RBC) normal metabolism and investigate the functional changes of red blood cells in the preservation process.

**Methods:** The methods are (1) the use of discontinuous density gradient separation to divide the whole blood into different fractions; (2) the use of spectrophotometry and flow cytometry determinated red blood age; (3) the use of flow cytometry, erythrocyte rosette test, and spectrophotometry detected red blood cell function; (4) exploration of the condition of in vitro RBC oxygen-carrying assay system and analysis of the change of RBC during preservation; and (5) in vivo, the changes of hemoglobin concentration after RBCs stored for variable time were transfused to β-thalassemia major (TM) patients have been studied.

**Results:** PS expression increased gradually with the increase of cell age and PK expression reversed. The positive rate of erythrocyte CR1 receptor expression and the number of CD35+ reduced with the cell age. *Q* value, P50, 2,3-DPG, and $Na^+$-$K^+$-ATPase gradually declined with the preservation time.

**Conclusion:** There is a close correlation between the red blood cell density and the age.

**Keywords:** red blood cell, transfusion, cell age, storage, function, dose

## 1. Introduction

Transfusion is important in clinical treatment, while red blood cell (RBC) is one of the most widely used components in transfusion medicine, but the function of RBC changed during their preservation as RBC storage lesion. Therefore, calculating the function dose of different storage time RBCs can achieve quantitative RBC transfusion, and improve the therapeutic effect of RBC transfusion. Here is the brief introduction to RBC transfusion and function dose as follows.

## 2. Focus of red blood cell transfusion research

### 2.1. Constant updating of red blood cell transfusion guidelines

A scientific reasonable blood transfusion can cure diseases and save lives, but as a coin has two sides, blood transfusion may bring transfusion risks. Blood transfusion cannot only transmit infectious diseases but also may give rise to hemolytic transfusion risk, as well as "Class III risk" [1]—anaphylactic reaction, transfusion-associated graft versus host disease (TA-GvHD), transfusion-related acute lung injury [2] (TRALI), transfusion-related immune modulation (TRIM), etc.

As an effective therapeutic measure for improving oxygen-carrying capacity and tissue hypoxia of anemia patients during clinical treatment, red blood cell (RBC) transfusion is being extensively applied clinically. There are various blood group antigens on RBC surface; thus transfused RBCs may bring hemolytic transfusion risks. According to statistics, the amount of transfusion is about 85 × 106U RBCs around the world every year [3]; however, RBC transfusion criteria vary with countries in RBC transfusion practice; one of the primary reasons may be the lack of high-quality evidence of advantages and disadvantages arising from RBC transfusion, so it is difficult to reach a consensus about RBC transfusion criteria. With deeper understanding of transfusion-related adverse reactions in clinical practice and increasingly significant blood supply versus demand contradiction, efficacy and safety of transfusion of stored RBCs become a problem to be addressed urgently in clinical transfusion practice.

"Red Blood Cell Transfusion Guidelines" [4] issued by American Association of Blood Banks (AABB) in 2012 proposed the recommendations of restrictive blood transfusion strategies and RBC transfusion criteria for adults and children with stable hemodynamics, in which RBC transfusion should be decided depending on patient symptoms and hemoglobin (Hb) level together. During the systematic retrospective analysis, no clinical study on transfusion threshold assessment for patients with acute coronary syndrome was found; therefore no recommendation can be given due to lack of clinical randomized controlled trial (RCT).

In October 2016, the latest version of "Red Blood Cell Transfusion Guidelines" was issued by AABB, aimed at establishing criteria for blood storage and transfusion behavior. Comparative study of restricted transfusion threshold and free transfusion threshold on 31 clinical trials from clinical randomized controlled trials with quantitative study hemoglobin threshold for RBC transfusion from 1950 to May 2016 revealed that the proportion of poor prognosis was not increased. Meanwhile 13 RCTs of 5515 patients subjected to random transfusion of fresh or stored RBC suspension from 1948 to May 2016 were compared, and it was found that fresh RBCs could not improve clinical prognosis. Furthermore, evidence-based advice for transfusion safety in terms of Hb level and RBC preservation time during RBC transfusion for most hemodynamically stable hospitalized adult patients was raised through Grading of Recommendations Assessment, Development and Evaluation (GRDE) study. Therefore, two Hb levels were set as transfusion thresholds in the recommendations: the restrictive RBC transfusion threshold for adult patients with stable hemodynamics, including severe patients, is 7 g/dL; for patients with past cardiovascular disease or patients subjected to cardiac or orthopedic surgery, the restrictive RBC transfusion threshold is 8 g/dL. The guidelines also demonstrate equal safety for most hospitalized patients in stable condition (even including neonates) to transfuse both stored RBCs within the validity period and stored blood within 10 days.

As can be seen from updates and advances of blood transfusion guidelines in recent years, RBC transfusion criteria have been changed from open strategy to restrictive strategy, and it has to further evolve to individualized transfusion strategy. In other words, RBC transfusion decision should not only rely on Hb level of a patient but also consider other factors, such as oxygen supply-associated symptoms and vital sign of patient individual and application of alternative blood transfusion protocol [5].

Although the Blood Transfusion Guidelines, issued by AABB in 2016, validate current restrictive transfusion strategy based on more randomized controlled studies of RBC transfusion and recommend two restrictive transfusion thresholds applicable to most patients in most cases so that blood transfusion decision becomes more individualized [6], the guidelines are still primarily limited in that setting blood transfusion threshold based on Hb level fails to consider fully other factors of oxygen supply balance and neither quantitates or semi-quantitates medical condition of a patient nor sets out a target Hb level of RBC transfusion; therefore, transfusion time and amount still rely more on clinical experience. And the new guidelines are applicable to most patients in perioperative period, critically ill patients with normal volume anemia, and internal medicine and geriatric patients. However, acute hemorrhage patients, patients with unstable hemodynamics, or selective operation patients with very low hemoglobin level due to acute massive hemorrhage are excluded. For patients with acute coronary syndrome, serious thrombocytopenia, and transfusion-dependent chronic anemia, no recommendation was made because of insufficient evidence.

### 2.2. Fresh RBCs and stored RBCs transfusion

RBC preservation time is a hot issue debated a lot in blood transfusion field; there are more than 50 observational studies reported about it [7, 8]. Most clinical transfusion researches discuss about effects of transfusion of "fresh" and "stored" RBCs on clinical prognosis of blood recipients. As the most common blood component, RBCs are one of the most widely used ingredients with the largest amount in transfusion therapy. The amount of blood collected worldwide each year exceeds 1 × 108 U. For preservative solutions ranging from sodium citrate, ACD, and CPD to CPDA and SAGM in popular application, RBC preservation time extends from the initial 5 to 42 days; nonetheless, a preservative solution can only delay aging of ex vivo RBCs, but cannot prevent its own aging process; therefore, as preservation time proceeds and metabolite accumulates [9], RBCs will change in shape and aggregation property, reduced oxygen-carrying capacity, and increased immunogenicity; changes of RBCs in oxygen-carrying capacity and immune functions are called "storage injuries" [10]. Current FDA standard allows frozen RBCs to be stored for up to 42 days prior to blood transfusion and stipulates that stored RBCs can be transfused back only after meeting two criteria as follows: (1) hemolytic rate of RBCs is less than 1% and (2) within 24 h after infusion, more than 75% of the red blood cells can survive in the body [11]. But more and more evidences demonstrate that, even if the above criteria are met, transfusion of RBCs which stored for a long time may still increase patient's risk of transfusion-associated adverse complications.

A large number of retrospective clinical studies show that transfusion of stored RBCs is associated with increased risk of cardiovascular events and higher mortality of clinically critical patients [11–13]; it is found in a study of cardiac surgery patients that, compared with patients who receive transfusion of stored RBCs alone or both fresh and stored RBCs, the fresh RBC transfusion group had a significantly decreased postoperative length of stay (PLOS). Among patients who receive transfusion of 1 URBCs, PLOS of patients receiving stored blood transfusion was 3.8 times more than that of patients receiving transfusion of fresh blood alone [14]. Nevertheless, this finding is still controversial. Lelubre and Vincent [15] conducted a systematic evaluation of such papers, which searched from MEDLINE covering a period from 1983 to December 2012, and studied the relevance of RBC preservation time to mortality or morbidity of adult patients. And they did not find any explicit argument to support superiority of fresh RBC transfusion (4 days) to stored RBC transfusion (26.5 days) in this systematic evaluation. Through the investigation of 1153 cardiac surgery patients with perioperative blood transfusion, McKenny et al. [16] also found that postoperative mortality, pulmonary infectious complication, ICU admission time, and postoperative ventilation duration were relevant to transfusion volume but irrelevant to blood preservation time. In 2015, the New England Journal of Medicine (NEJM) published a multicenter randomized clinical trial with important reference value [17], showing that, with 90-day mortality as primary outcome measure, disease outcomes were not statistically different between critically ill patients who received transfusion of fresh RBCs stored for up to 10 days ($6.1 \pm 4.9$ days) and critically ill patients who received transfusion of stored RBC (storage time, $22 \pm 8.4$ days) in line with "first-in-first-out" principle, and between-group comparisons in secondary outcome measures (main complications, respiration, hemodynamics, renal support treatment duration, length of stay, and transfusion reaction incidence) and comparisons between subgroups (age, APACHE score, number of transfused RBC units, disease type such as medicine, surgery, and injury) show no statistical difference. In the same year, NEJM reported that Steiner et al. performed a prospective multicenter randomized study of cardiac surgery patients [18], finding that even if storage time was longer than 21 days, prognosis of transfusion recipients would not be affected. It is found that comparison between transfusion of fresh RBCs (<10 days) and transfusion of RBCs having a storage period >21 days show no significant difference in adverse events, except high probability of hyperbilirubinemia occurring in the long-term storage group. In a trial of 377 extremely low birth weight neonates and preterm infants who received randomly fresh RBCs (<8 days) or stored RBCs [19], adverse outcome incidence had no difference between groups. Heddle's observational study [20] also suggested that, in general, nosocomial mortality of hospitalized patients was irrelevant to storage time of transfused RBCs, but this study failed to observe transfusion of old RBCs having a storage time of 35–42 days [21], so it is biased. Dhabangi and Fergusson et al. [22, 23] did not find any difference in clinical prognosis between transfusion of RBCs having a storage time of 21–28 days and transfusion of RBCs having a storage time <7 days. The Blood Transfusion Guidelines issued by AABB in 2016 strongly recommended that RBCs at any time within storage period can be transfused into hospitalized patients including neonates, based on evidence that fresh RBCs (stored for <10 days) and RBCs within standard storage period are transfused in most RCT samples, whereas only a very few samples receive transfusion of old RBCs having a storage time of 36–42 days. The National Blood Collection and Utilization Survey Report issued by the US Department of Health and Human Services (US DHHS) pointed out that RBCs transfused in the USA had mean storage duration of 17.9 days, so the AABB guidelines did not assess RBCs stored for more than 35 days, either. Unexpectedly, The Lancet published a retrospective cohort study in 2016 [24], in which the investigators divided 91,065 transfusion events (all RBCs were leukofiltered) occurring in 23,634 adult patients during 2008–2014 into fresh RBC group (1–7 days), mid-term RBC group (3–5 days), and long-term RBC group (36–42 days) by RBC storage time, assessed effects of blood storage time on a 90-day mortality of transfusion recipients and concluded that overall mortality risk of fresh RBC group was higher than that of long-term RBC group and a 90-day mortality of patients receiving transfusion of fresh RBCs was higher than those of patients receiving transfusion of stored RBCs; the research team said that its causes had to be further studied.

We can find from a number of observational (retrospective and prospective) study reports that transfusion of RBCs having average blood storage times differing by more than 10 days was mostly studied, though the dividing time point between fresh RBCs and stored RBCs has not yet been uniformly defined; meanwhile, due to scarcity of blood resource, patients seldom receive transfusion of old RBCs (>35 days) in clinical practice, which enables the presence of multiple independent confounding variables that may influence outcome measures in RCT studies and clinical trials, such as site (treatment difference), disease severity, transfusion occurring after a clinical event, etc., all of which will cause biases. Therefore, research that lacks multicenter and large-sample randomized controlled data cannot help one assess correctly benefits and hazards of intervention measures [24]. Importantly, none of the studies clarified that transfusion of stored RBCs would cause any harm in clinical transfusion [7, 25].

### 2.3. Open transfusion strategy and restrictive transfusion strategy

RBC transfusion plays an irreplaceable important role in correcting anemia and surgical and trauma ischemia rescue. Upon anemia, Hb level falls, blood viscosity declines, blood flow volume increases, and 2,3-DPG activity is stronger, so that tissue blood flow volume and oxygen release increase [26], not only lowering tissue (including myocardium) oxygen supply but also needing higher cardiac output to maintain sufficient systemic oxygen supply so as to meet myocardial oxygen demand; therefore RBC transfusion becomes an effective treatment mode for full restoration of tissue oxygen supply in the event of insufficient oxygen supply [27]. Given that anemia is closely related to preoperative anemia or poor prognosis of cardiovascular disease [28], most clinicians select free transfusion strategy based on clinical experience; however, when most patients are hemodynamically stable, hemoglobin threshold of ordinary critically care patients [29] is 7 g/dL; patients having Hb level of 7–9 g/dL did not need blood transfusion, unless there is any particular comorbidity or acute disease-related factor changed clinical decision. Initially, RBC transfusion used to adopt open transfusion strategy or use higher Hb level to trigger blood transfusion. Adams and Lundy proposed initially "10/30 criterion" in 1942 [30], that is, blood is transfused when Hb level declines below 10 g/dL or hematocrit (Hct) falls below 30%, which has served as a trigger of RBC transfusion in decades though there is a paucity of clinical evidence [27]. From updates and advances of blood transfusion guidelines and blood transfusion indications in the past years, we can see that RBC transfusion indications have gradually transformed from open transfusion strategy to restrictive transfusion strategy in clinical transfusion practice; the Blood Transfusion Guidelines updated by AABB in 2016 also support restrictive transfusion strategy with large-scale multicenter RCT evidence without increasing incidence rate of adverse clinical outcome.

In recent years, a large amount of data of many RCTs studying clinical influences of transfusion strategies support more and more vigorous RBC transfusion strategy. In terms of clinical therapeutic effect, restrictive RBC transfusion strategy is at least not inferior to or even superior to open RBC transfusion strategy. For people receiving surgery or critical care, the restrictive transfusion strategy has been proven to be safe and even safer than free transfusion strategy in some cases. In a prospective RCT conducted by Hajjar et al. [31], during hospitalization of adult patients receiving cardiac surgery with extracorporeal circulation, differences of 30-day mortality and severe morbidity (cardiogenic shock, acute respiratory distress syndrome, or acute kidney injury necessitating renal dialysis or hemodialysis) between free transfusion strategy group and restricted transfusion strategy group were not statistically significant. In 2011, the New England Journal of Medicine reported that [32], for high cardiovascular-risk patients aged above 50 under hip surgery, starting blood transfusion at a Hb level of 100 g/L did not yield a lower mortality or hospitalized morbidity than starting blood transfusion at 80 g/L. For adult acute leukemia patients under chemotherapy [33], restrictive transfusion strategy had no impact on 30–100-day mortality, hemorrhage, and length of stay. To determine hemoglobin threshold of patients with acute gastroenteric hemorrhage, investigators recruited 921 patients with acute upper gastrointestinal hemorrhage, assigned transfusion strategy at random, and stratified the subjects depending on whether or not a subject contracts liver cirrhosis, finding that restrictive transfusion strategy improved significantly prognosis of patients with acute upper gastrointestinal hemorrhage, as compared with free transfusion strategy [34], which agrees with the finding of previous observational study and RCT that restrictive transfusion strategy did not increase [32] but even decreased [35] mortality. As shown in a study [36], the use of restrictive hemoglobin threshold enabled RBC transfusion rate to fall by 43%, and compared with free transfusion strategy, no evidence indicated that the restrictive transfusion strategy affected a 30-day mortality; the researchers further assessed other adverse clinical prognoses, including infection (pneumonia, wound infection, and sepsis), heart disease, apoplexy, and thrombosis and did not find any difference between both transfusion strategies, either. Therefore, we can know that, for hemodynamically stable hospitalized patients, restrictive transfusion strategy (7–8 g/dL) is at least effective like free transfusion strategy (hemoglobin threshold, 7–10 g/dL) and does not produce any result adverse to clinical prognosis, including a 30-day mortality, cardiac morbidity, and infection. In other words, no RCT data can verify that higher hemoglobin threshold (9–10 g/dL) will benefit clinical prognosis. In addition, a single-center RCT conducted by Shehata et al. [37] also demonstrated that, for high-risk heart disease patients who adopted randomly restricted transfusion strategy or open transfusion strategy, between-group comparison shows no difference in individual adverse prognosis. Therefore, triggering blood transfusion in strict accordance with restrictive hemoglobin threshold in clinical transfusion practice would decrease greatly transfusion volume of a patient and could lower unnecessary blood transfusion risk of the patient. Rohde et al. [38] made a systematic review of clinical RCT data of hospitalized patients involving RBC transfusion threshold and ran meta-analysis of relevance of restrictive and free RBC transfusion strategies to medical infection, and the results indicate that restrictive transfusion strategy is irrelevant to holistic medicine-associated infection reduction, but restrictive RBC transfusion strategy is relevant to reduction in serious infection risk.

The transfusion should be started with one unit of RBCs rather than two in clinical transfusion practice when following the restrictive transfusion strategy; this may have important impact on blood transfusion behavior. Moreover, development of blood protection measures also enriches connotation of the restrictive transfusion strategy, so as to attain no or less blood transfusion. Blood protection measures include certainty of blood transfusion indications, treating anemia with iron supplement, minimizing the use of ischemia drugs, using autologous blood transfusion to patients with large blood loss, etc.

## 3. Functional dose of RBC

### 3.1. Concept of RBC "functional dose"

The main functions of RBCs consist of oxygen-carrying function and immune functions. Oxygen-carrying function of mature RBCs is evaluated worldwide by using many methods: P50, 2,3-DPG, effective oxygen-carrying capacity (*Q*), and $Na^+$-$K^+$-ATPase. The most primary immune function of RBCs is to remove circulating immune complexes (CICs); the complement C3b receptor (CR1) on membrane surface is able to adhere to and bind CICs in blood, bring them to mononuclear phagocyte systems of the liver and spleen, and then dissociate and remove them, so as to reduce CIC deposition in tissues. Therefore, quantitative assay of CR1 molecules in RBCs and quantitative evaluation of their bioactivity can help assess immune function state of RBCs at different days of age.

So far the quality standards of suspended RBC mainly focused on RBC count and hemolytic change during the preservation; however, the stored RBC in the preservation period could experience the aging process of RBC itself on one hand; on the other hand, RBC oxygen-carrying function and immune function will change due to damage of RBC in preservation. Following the prolonging of preservation time of RBC, aging RBC will increase concurrently, while the cell volume will decrease, hemoglobin content will decrease, cell density will increase, the activity of pyruvate kinase (PK) will decrease, P50 will decrease significantly, RBC oxygen affinity will increase [39], and RBC oxygen-binding ability gets stronger, which is not conducive to oxygen release. At the same time, the level of C3b is decreased, which gives rise to the apparent weakening of its immune adherence function as well as the capacity to clear the pathological circulating immune complex. Therefore, the amount of RBC used in the present situation as well as oxygen-carrying function cannot accurately reflect the true situation of RBC. However, the function of storing RBCs and fresh RBCs was regarded as the same in clinical at present. It is reported that storage damages of red blood cells in vitro and at low temperature can reduce the deformability of red blood cells, 2,3-DPG, and oxygen-carrying capacity which lead to reduction of infusion efficiency [40]. In order to accurately reflect the functional status of RBC at different preservation time, we proposed that the dose unit of RBC should use the "functional dose" unit. "Functional dose" of 1 RBC refers to the function of the RBC contained in 200 mL whole blood under physiological conditions (oxygen-carrying capacity and immunity).

### 3.2. Study on the days of age and function of mature RBC under physiological conditions

The average life expectancy of mature RBC in healthy adults is about 115–120 days [41]; RBCs are constantly emerging and damaged, which maintain a dynamic balance. Adults need to update 200 billion (2 × 1012) RBC per day to maintain the total amount of 2–3 × 1013 RBC in the body [42]. Therefore, the RBC in the body is a heterogeneous group of RBC with different days of age.

Based on the change of red blood cell density, Wu Zhou et al. from our laboratory [43] divided the whole blood RBCs into six different density gradients by discontinuous density gradient separation method at low temperature and low centrifugal force within a short time and then detected the ratio of pyruvate kinase of each layer of RBC and pyruvate kinase activity in RBC of whole blood, days of age of RBC were calculated according to Bracey on the RBC pyruvate kinase ratio and the average age of the RBC data, different density of RBC represent RBC of different days of age, and the correlation between RBC density and its days of age was revealed according to the expression positive age of phosphatidylserine on the surface layers of RBC membrane; the quantitative measurement of CRI molecules and the quantitative evaluation of its bioactivity were conducted to evaluate the immune function of RBC of different days of age, the natural immune adhesion tumor cell rosette test was used to detect immune activity of RBC immune activity, and the method of measuring the oxygen-carrying capacity of RBC was discussed.

#### *3.2.1. Isolating RBC populations with variable days of age by discontinuous density gradient method.*

As shown in **Figure 1** courtesy of *Wu Zhou*, centrifuging RBCs at 3500 g and 10 °C for 20 min yielded six clearly stratified density layers, and their average RBC days of age (in the ascending order of density) could be obtained from ratio values and the calculation formula for average RBC days age: 11.5, 46, 63.8, 74.6, 80.5, and 102.2.

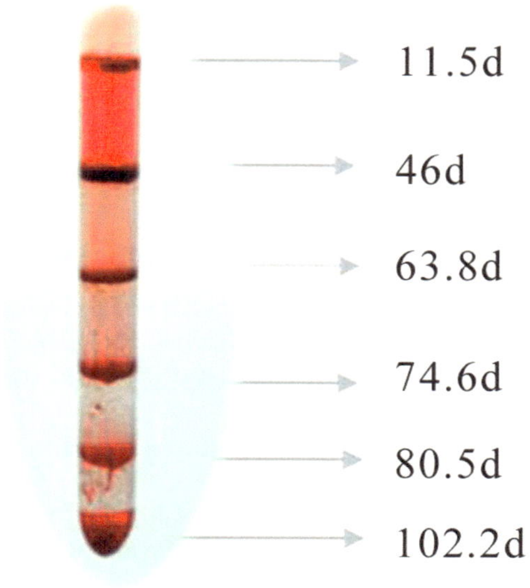


**Figure 1.** Different ages of red blood cell separation.

*3.2.2. Assay of pyruvate kinase activity*

**Table 1** lists ratios of pyruvate kinase (PK) activity of stratified RBCs at different density to that of the whole blood, from low-density portion (layer 1) to high-density portion (layer 6); PK activity weakened gradually and phosphatidylserine (PS) expression increased gradually. According to ratio formula, ratio = PK activity of stratified RBCs with variable density/ PK activity of non-isolated RBCs (whole blood), days of age of RBCs with variable density in **Figure 1** were calculated.

| Cell stratification | PK (U/gHb) | PK (Ratio) | $PS^+$ (%) |
|---|---|---|---|
| Whole blood | 5.62 ± 1.15 | | 0.73 ± 0.46 |
| 1 | 8.11 ± 1.70 | 1.49 ± 0.44 | 0.36 ± 0.16 |
| 2 | 6.21 ± 1.24* | 1.14 ± 0.32 | 0.53 ± 0.24 |
| 3 | 5.16 ± 1.23* | 0.96 ± 0.31 | 0.59 ± 0.12 |
| 4 | 4.53 ± 1.06*, # | 0.85 ± 0.26 | 0.67 ± 0.21 |
| 5 | 4.37 ± 0.68*, # | 0.79 ± 0.13 | 0.61 ± 0.19 |
| 6 | 3.20 ± 0.74*, #, △ | 0.57 ± 0.11 | 1.03 ± 0.88* |

*Compare with the first layer, $P < 0.05$.
#Compare with the second layer, $P < 0.05$.
△Compare with the third layer, $P < 0.05 (n = 10)$.

**Table 1.** Erythrocyte PK activity and the ratio of PK activity to the whole blood.

*3.2.3. Study on days of age versus function for mature RBCs under physiological condition*

Difference in number of CD35 (CR1 receptor) molecules shown between RBC populations at different days of age is just one manifestation of immune function difference shown in process of RBC aging, while innate immune adherence rosette test is just one aspect of RBC receptor immunoactivity. As shown in **Figure 2**, the higher the RBC density, the fewer the RBCs with positively expressed CD35 molecules, and the lower the immune adherence rosette rate of different stratified cells, and the rosette rate declined more significantly than CD35 RBC percentage.

Mature RBC age in physiological state and oxygen-carrying function is shown in **Figure 3**. As shown in **Figure 3**, RBCs at different days of age differed significantly in oxygen-carrying capacity, and RBC function was inversely correlated with RBC days of age.

### 3.3. Regulated changes of RBC function under storage condition

It is well known that RBCs will change in morphology and function during storage: RBC volume is getting smaller, and RBC density is increasing, relating to RBC aging associated with cell membrane vesiculation [44], resulting in loss of cell membrane and some intracellular hemoglobin and weakened regulating capacity of supramembrane $Na^+$-$K^+$ ion pump. RBC transfusion in stored state cannot improve an organism's capability of taking in oxygen, which is associated with reduction in oxygen-carrying capacity of stored RBCs [45]. Such reduction is even earlier than reduction in 2,3-DPG [45, 46]. Therefore, measured *Q* value, 2,3-DPG, P50, and $Na^+$-$K^+$-ATPase of stored blood can be used to evaluate effects of blood stored for different times on oxygen-carrying function of RBCs [46]. Then, how will oxygen-carrying capacity of RBCs change with variable storage time? Is transfusion of stored RBCs further capable of supplying oxygen to organism tissues very efficiently? How is RBC transfusion volume determined to

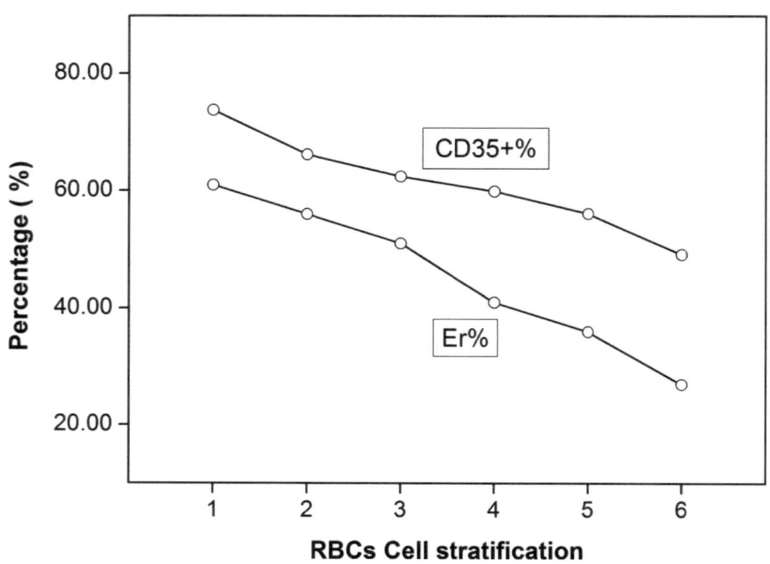


**Figure 2.** Changes in immune functions of various ages of RBC under physiological conditions.

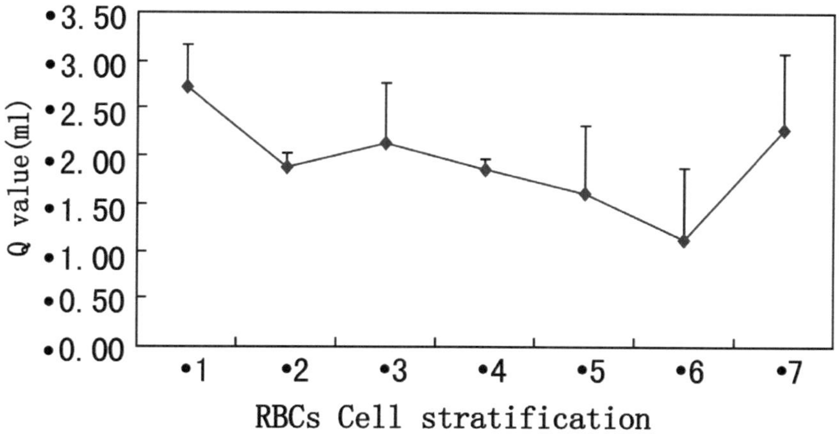


**Figure 3.** Different ages of RBCs and $Q$ changes under physiological status. Note: 7 is not separated before the whole blood specimens.

achieve the same treatment effect? Can we quantitate oxygen-carrying capacity of stored RBCs to provide transfusion dose to clinical transfusion more accurately?

In 2013, Ting et al. [47] conducted a study on oxygen-carrying capacity of RBC in different storage time and obtained the change law of oxygen-carrying capacity of RBC suspension at different ages. As shown in **Figures 4–7**, the values of $Q$ and P50 were decreased with the increase of the number of days during storage, among which the faster decrease appeared in the first 14 days. With the concentration of 2,3-DPG was decreased gradually, it was difficult to release $O_2$, ATPase decreased with the increase of storage time, and the most severe decrease appeared in the first 7 days. It can be seen that in a full linear correlation between $Q$ value and P50, the oxygen-carrying capacity of RBCs depends on their own aging variation. The authors established a mathematical multivariate linear model, with effective oxygen-carrying volume as the dependent variable and 2,3-DPG, $Na^+$-$K^+$-ATPase, and storage time as independent variables: the multivariate linear model was $Q = 5.457 - 0.925 \times$ 2,3-DPG + $0.142 \times Na^+$-$K^+$-ATPase $-0.076 \times T$ (Storage days), and we obtained functional doses of RBCs stored in vitro for different days. Physical packaging dose unit fails to effectively reflect functions of RBCs transfused at various time points during storage period; therefore establishing a conversion formula for determining oxygen-carrying capacity coefficient of unit RBC stored for different days can enable realistic quantitative transfusion, guide clinical blood use with scientific functional dose, and improve RBC treatment effect.

### 3.4. Functional dose of RBCs for clinical trial

Based on the above in vitro RBC tests, we found that oxygen-carrying capacity of RBCs declined progressively with increasing storage time. In order to explore clinical transfusion efficacy of RBCs versus storage time and provide experimental data for quantitative transfusion of RBCs, Yunayuan et al. [48] observed changes of hemoglobin concentration after RBCs stored for variable time were transfused to β-thalassemia major (TM) patients. The authors collected 52 (persons) parts (400 mL/part) of blood that were leukofiltered within 6–8 h, had

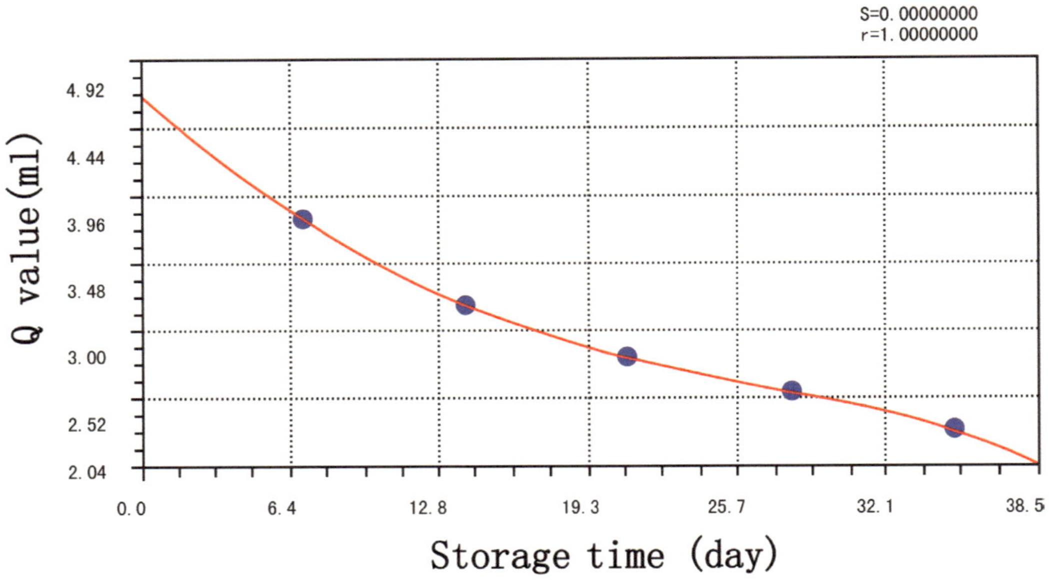


**Figure 4.** Changes of *Q* value of red blood cells in stock of different ages.

a RBC Hct of 45–47% and passed routine inspection, then divided each part into two aliquots of 1 U (200 mL/U) leukoreduced RBCs for later use; leukoreduced RBCs that were collected from one same blood donor and stored until Day 3 (fresh blood, 1U) and Day 17 (old blood, 1U) were transfused into 52 TM patients enrolled as per study criteria; blood routine, blood gas analysis, and 2,3-DGP concentration were assayed 24 h prior to and 24 h after transfusion

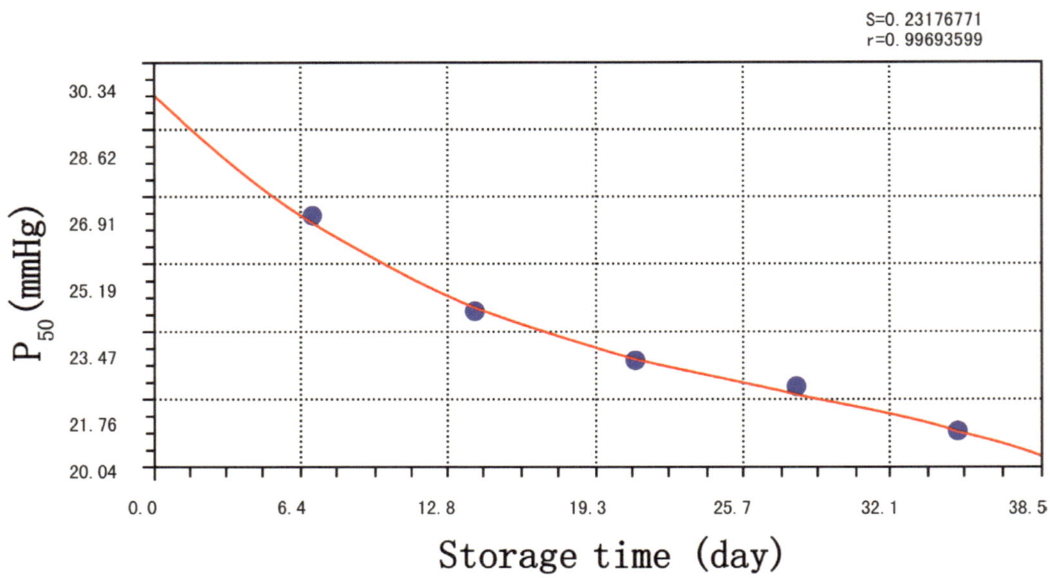


**Figure 5.** Changes of P50 of red blood cells in stock of different ages.

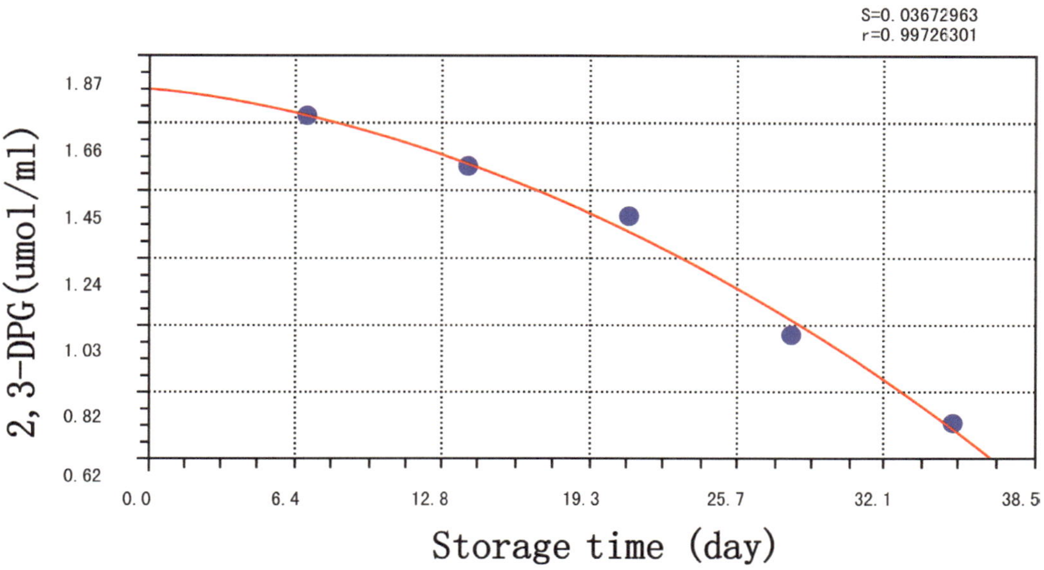


**Figure 6.** Changes of 2,3-DPG of red blood cells in stock of different ages.

and on day 14 after transfusion, respectively. Variations per 10 kg of body weight 24 h and 14 days after every transfusion were compared. In the trial, there are 10 dropout cases and 42 completed cases. The results are shown in **Figures 8** and **9**: Hb and 2,3-DGP of patients receiving transfusion of blood stored for 3 days were obviously better than those of patients receiving transfusion of blood stored for 17 days.

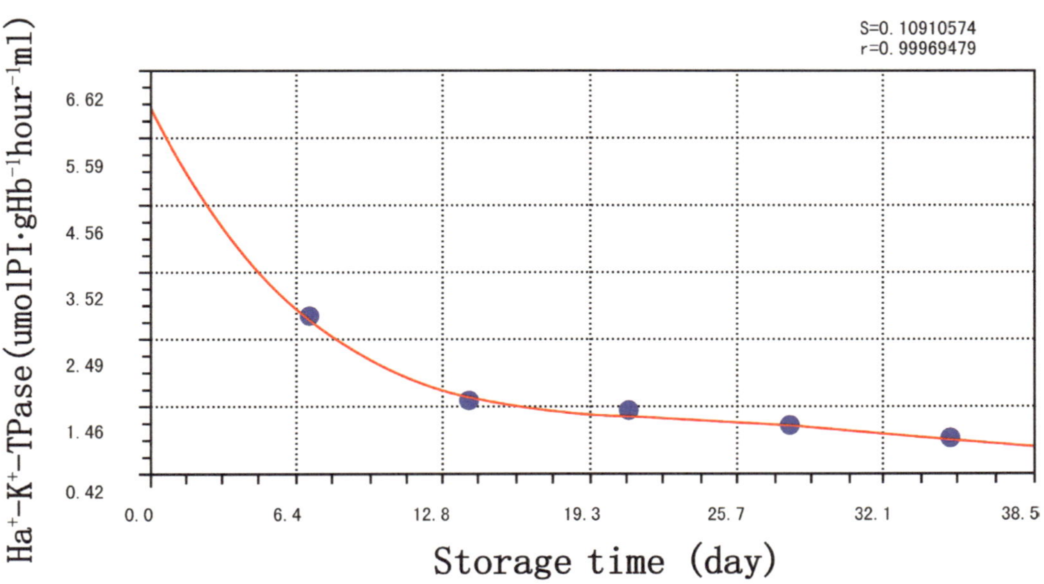


**Figure 7.** Changes of $Na^{+}$-$K^{+}$-ATPase of red blood cells in stock of different ages.

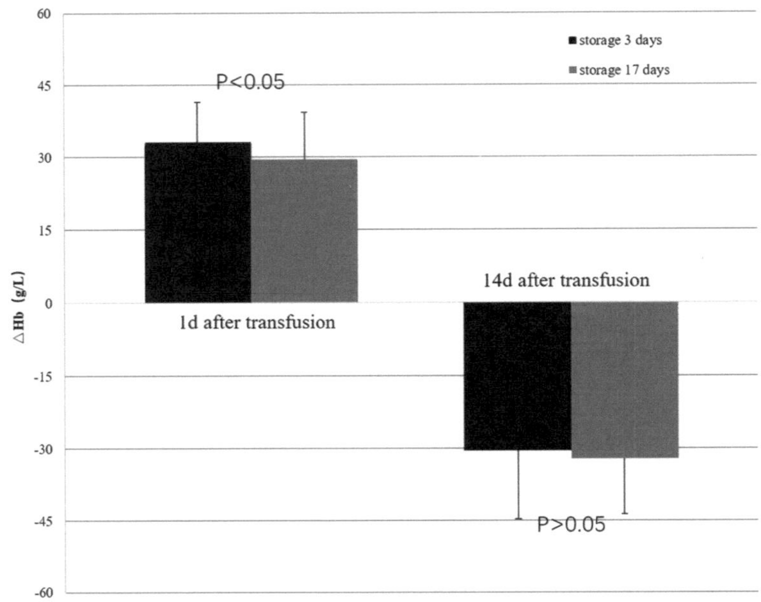


**Figure 8.** Different storage times of RBC transfusion in patients with Hb changes. $n = 42$.

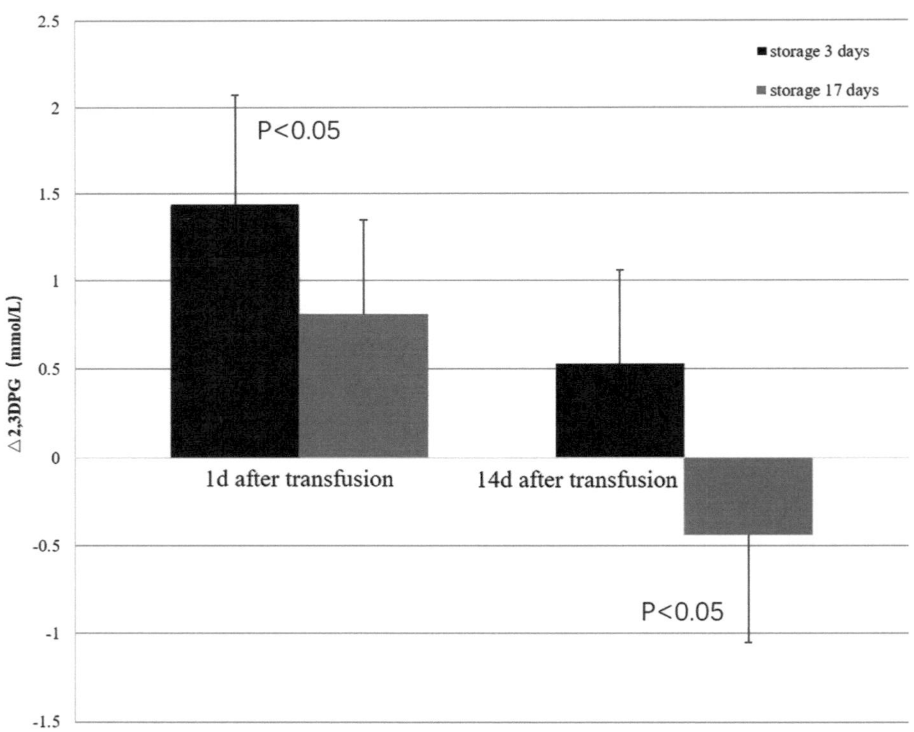


**Figure 9.** Different storage times of RBC transfusion in patients with 2,3-DGP changes. $n = 42$.

## 4. Conclusion

Blood transfusion has an irreplaceable position and significance in rescuing patients, and the blood belongs to the scarce resource because of the long-time shortage worldwide. In light of this situation, it is most necessary to have a good command of transfusion indications in clinical transfusion practice, determine the optimum therapeutic dose, and supply safe and effective blood within storage period for rescue treatment of patients. After functional doses of RBCs with different storage times are determined, quantitative RBC transfusion can be achieved to minimize transfusion risk and improve RBC transfusion efficacy, which is the ultimate objective of our study.

## Acknowledgements

On the completion of my paper, I would like to express my deepest gratitude to all whose kindness and advice have made this work possible. We thank my Master student Wu Zhou and Ting Zhang who completed the basic and clinical trials of the red blood cell functional dose and provided the experimental data. We thank Yunayuan He for supporting the clinical trial data.

## Author details

Deqing Wang* and Leiying Zhang

*Address all correspondence to: deqingwang@vip.sina.com

Department of Blood Transfusion, Chinese PLA General Hospital, Beijing, China

## References

[1] Fengyan F, Deqing W. Transfusion risk understanding process change – Discussion on the third kind of blood transfusion risk. Journal of Clinical Transfusion and Laboratory Medicine. 2016;**18**(1):1-4

[2] Delaney M, Wendel S, Bercovitz RS, Biomedical Excellence for Safer Transfusion (BEST) Collaborative. Transfusion reactions: Prevention, diagnosis, and treatment. Lancet. 2016;**388**(10061):2825-2836. DOI: 10.1016/S0140-6736(15)01313-6

[3] Takei T, Amin NA, Schmid G. Progress in global blood safety for HIV. Journal of Acquired Immune Deficiency Syndromes. 2009;**52**(Suppl 2):S127-S131. DOI: 10.1097/QAI.0b013e3181baf0ac

[4] Carson JL, Grossman BJ, Kleinman S. Red blood cell transfusion: A clinical practice guideline from the AABB*. Annals of Internal Medicine. 2012;**157**(1):49-58. DOI: 10.7326/0003-4819-157-1-201206190-00429

[5] Padhi S, Kemmis-Betty S, Rajesh S. Blood transfusion: Summary of NICE guidance. British Medical Journal 2015;**351**:h5832. DOI: 10.1136/bmj.h5832. No abstract available

[6] Yazer MH, Triulzi DJ. AABB red blood cell transfusion guidelines: Something for almost everyone. Journal of the American Medical Association. 2016;**316**(19):1984-1985. DOI: 10.1001/jama.2016.10887

[7] van de Watering LM. Age of blood: Does older blood yield poorer outcomes? Current Opinion in Hematology. 2013;**20**(6):526-532. DOI: 10.1097/MOH.0b013e328365aa3a

[8] Remy KE, Sun J, Wang D. Transfusion of recently donated (fresh) red blood cells (RBCs) does not improve survival in comparison with current practice, while safety of the oldest stored units is yet to be established: A meta-analysis. Vox Sanguinis. 2016;**111**(1):43-54. DOI: 10.1111/vox.12380. Epub 2016 Feb 5

[9] Aubron C, Nichol A, Cooper DJ. Age of red blood cells and transfusion in critically ill patients. Annals of Intensive Care. 2013;**3**(1):2. DOI: 10.1186/2110-5820-3-2

[10] Bennett-Guerrero E, Veldman TH, Doctor A. Evolution of adverse changes in stored RBCs. Proceedings of the National Academy of Sciences of the United States of America. 2007;**104**(43):17063-17068. DOI: 10.1073/pnas.0708160104

[11] Triulzi DJ, Yazer MH. Clinical studies of the effect of blood storage on patient outcomes. Transfusion and Apheresis Science. 2010;**43**(1):95-106. DOI: 10.1016/j.transci.2010.05.013

[12] Wang D, Sun J, Solomon SB. Transfusion of older stored blood and risk of death: A meta-analysis. Transfusion. 2012;**52**(6):1184-1195

[13] Pettilä V, Westbrook AJ, Nichol AD. Age of red blood cells and mortality in the critically ill. Critical Care. 2011;**15**(2):R116. DOI: 10.1186/cc10142

[14] Sanders J, Patel S, Cooper J. Red blood cell storage is associated with length of stay and renal complications after cardiac surgery. Transfusion. 2011;**51**(11):2286-2294. DOI: 10.1111/j.1537-2995.2011.03170.x

[15] Lelubre C, Vincent JL. Relationship between red cell storage duration and outcomes in adults receiving red cell transfusions: A systematic review. Critical Care. 2013;**17**(2):R66. DOI: 10.1186/cc12600

[16] McKenny M, Ryan T, Tate H. Age of transfused blood is not associated with increased postoperative adverse outcome after cardiac surgery. British Journal of Anaesthesia. 2011;**106**(5):643-649. DOI: 10.1093/bja/aer029

[17] Lacroix J, Hebert PC, Fergusson DA. Age of transfused blood in critically ill adults. New England Journal of Medicine. 2015;**372**:1410-1418. DOI: 10.1056/NEJMoa1500704

[18] Steiner ME, Ness PM, Assmann SF. Effects of red-cell storage duration on patients undergoing cardiac surgery. New England Journal of Medicine. 2015;**372**(15):1419-1429. DOI: 10.1056/NEJMoa1414219

[19] Fergusson DA, Hébert P, Hogan DL. Effect of fresh red blood cell transfusions on clinical outcomes in premature, very low-birth-weight infants: The ARIPI randomized trial. Journal of the American Medical Association. 2012;**308**(14):1443-1451. DOI: 10.1001/2012.jama.11953

[20] Heddle NM, Cook RJ, Arnold DM. Effect of short-term vs. long-term blood storage on mortality after transfusion. New England Journal of Medicine. 2016;**375**(20):1937-1945. DOI: 10.1056/NEJMoa1609014

[21] Klein HG, Cortés-Puch I, Natanson C. More on the age of transfused red cells. New England Journal of Medicine. 2015;**373**(3):283-284. DOI: 10.1056/NEJMc1505699#SA1

[22] Dhabangi A, Ainomugisha B, Cserti-Gazdewich C. Effect of transfusion of red blood cells with longer vs shorter storage duration on elevated blood lactate levels in children with severe anemia: The TOTAL randomized clinical trial. Journal of the American Medical Association. 2015;**314**(23):2514-2523. DOI: 10.1001/jama.2015.13977

[23] Fergusson D, Tinmouth A. Storage age of red blood cells for transfusion of premature infants-reply. Journal of the American Medical Association. 2013;**309**(6):545. DOI: 10.1001/jama.2012.177442

[24] Heddle NM, Arnold DM, Acker JP, et al. Red blood cell processing methods and in-hospital mortality: A transfusion registry cohort study. The Lancet Haematology. 2016;**3**(5):e246-e254. bian229. DOI: 10.1016/S2352-3026(16)00020-X

[25] Jakobsen JC, Gluud C. The necessity of randomized clinical trials. British Journal of Medicine & Medical Research. 2013;**3**(4):1453-1468

[26] Goodnough LT, Schrier SL. Evaluation and management of anemia in the elderly. American Journal of Hematology. 2014;**89**(1):88-96

[27] Wang JK, Klein HG. Red blood cell transfusion in the treatment and management of anaemia: The search for the elusive transfusion trigger. Vox Sanguinis. 2010;**98**(1):2-11. DOI: 10.1111/j.1423-0410.2009.01223.x

[28] Shander A, Javidroozi M, Naqvi S. An update on mortality and morbidity in patients with very low postoperative hemoglobin levels who decline blood transfusion (CME). Transfusion. 2014 Oct;**54**(10 Pt 2):2688-2695; quiz 2687. DOI: 10.1111/trf.12565

[29] Retter A, Wyncoll D, Pearse R. Guidelines on the management of anaemia and red cell transfusion in adult ill patients. British Journal of Haematology. 2013;**160**(4):445-464. DOI: 10.1111/bjh.12143

[30] Adams RC, Lundy JS. Anesthesia in cases of poor surgical risk: Some suggestions for decreasing the risk. Surgery, Gynecology & Obstetrics. 1942;**74**:1011-1019

[31] Hajjar LA, Vincent JL, Galas FR. Transfusion requirements after cardiac surgery: The TRACS randomized controlled trial. Journal of the American Medical Association. 2010;**304**(14):1559-1567. DOI: 10.1001/jama.2010.1446

[32] Carson JL, Terrin ML, Noveck H. Liberal or restrictive transfusion in high-risk patients after hip surgery. New England Journal of Medicine. 2011;**365**(26):2453-2462. DOI: 10.1056/NEJMoa1012452

[33] Estcourt LJ, Malouf R, Trivella M, et al. Restrictive versus liberal red blood cell transfusion strategies for people with haematological malignancies treated with intensive chemotherapy or radiotherapy, or both, with or without haematopoietic stem cell support. Cochrane Database Syst Rev. 2017 Jan 27; CD011305. DOI: 10.1002/14651858.CD011305.pub2

[34] Villanueva C, Colomo A, Bosch A. Transfusion strategies for acute upper gastrointestinal bleeding. New England Journal of Medicine. 2013;**368**(1):11-21. DOI: 10.1056/NEJMoa1211801

[35] Marik PE, Corwin HL. Efficacy of red blood cell transfusion in the critically ill: A systematic review of the literature. Critical Care Medicine. 2008;**36**(9):2667-2674. DOI: 10.1097/CCM.0b013e3181844677

[36] Carson JL, Stanworth SJ, Roubinian N. Transfusion thresholds and other strategies for guiding allogeneic red blood cell transfusion. The Cochrane Database of Systematic Reviews. 2016;**10**:CD002042. DOI: 10.1002/14651858.CD002042.pub4

[37] Shehata N, Burns LA, Nathan H. A randomized controlled pilot study of adherence to transfusion strategies in cardiac surgery. Transfusion. 2012;**52**(1):91-99. DOI: 10.1111/j.1537-2995.2011.03236.x

[38] Rohde JM, Dimcheff DE, Blumberg N. Health care-associated infection after red blood cell transfusion: A systematic review and meta-analysis. Journal of the American Medical Association. 2014;**311**(13):1317-1326. DOI: 10.1001/jama.2014.2726

[39] Gelderman MP, Yazer MH, Jia Y. Serial oxygen equilibrium and kinetic measurements during RBC storage. Transfusion Medicine. 2010;**20**(5):341-345. DOI: 10.1111/j.1365-3148.2010.01016.x

[40] Bonaventura J. Clinical implications of the loss of vasoactive nitric oxide during red blood cell storage. Proceedings of the National Academy of Sciences of the United States of America. 2007;**104**(49):19165-6. DOI: 10.1073/pnas.0708871105

[41] Rifkind JM, Nagababu E. Hemoglobin redox reactions and red blood cell aging. Antioxid Redox Signal. 2013;**18**(17):2274-2283. DOI: 10.1089/ars.2012.4867

[42] Palis J. Primitive and definitive erythropoiesis in mammals. Frontiers in Physiology. 2014;**5**:3. DOI: 10.3389/fphys.2014.00003

[43] Wu Z, Shuying W, Deqing W. Study on the relationship between red blood cell density and age. Chinese Journal of Blood Transfusion. 2011;**24**(2):113-115

[44] Antonelou MH, Kriebardis AG, Papassideri IS. Aging and death signalling in mature red cells: From basic science to transfusion practice. Blood Transfusion. 2010:**8** Suppl 3:s39-47. DOI: 10.2450/2010.007S

[45] Wei C, Yu Y, Chen Y. Impact of warming blood transfusion and infusion toward cerebral oxygen metabolism and cognitive recovery in the perioperative period of elderly knee replacement. Journal of Orthopaedic Surgery and Research. 2014;**10**:8

[46] Tinmouth A, Fergusson D, Yee IC. Clinical consequences of red cell storage in the critically ill. Transfusion. 2006 Nov;**46**(11):2014-2027. DOI: 10.1111/j.1537-2995.2006.01026.x

[47] Ting Z, Jichun P, Yuan Z. Changes of oxygen carrying capacity of red blood cells in different storage time. Chinese Journal of Blood Transfusion. 2013;**26**(5):420-424

[48] Yunayuan H, Lihong Z, Yuan Z. Changes of hemoglobin concentration in patients with severe beta thalassemia after different time of transfusion. Chinese Journal of Blood Transfusion. 2015;**11**(28):1351-1354

Chapter 6

# Transfusion in Transplantation

Eren Arslan Davulcu, Fahri Sahin and Güray Saydam

Additional information is available at the end of the chapter

http://dx.doi.org/10.5772/intechopen.69260

**Abstract**

Hematopoietic stem cell transplantation is increasingly performed in several diseases; majority of them are hematologic malignancies. Hematopoietic stem cell transplantation is not an instant procedure; contrarily, its unique clinical and laboratorial consequences may take life-long time. Blood product transfusion is an inevitable and critical component for the management. Hematopoietic stem cell transplant patients have different requirements regarding blood products transfusion because of their immune status, long-term cytopenias and especially HLA and ABO incompatibilities. Health-care staff who take a part in the management of those patients should be aware of specific and specialized transfusion requirements.

**Keywords:** transfusion, hematopoietic stem cell transplantation, allogeneic, autologous, blood products

## 1. Introduction

### 1.1. Definition of hematopoietic stem cell transplantation

Hematopoietic stem cell transplantation (HSCT) is the procedure that is transplantation of multipotent hematopoietic stem cells, which are derived from bone marrow, peripheral blood, or umbilical cord blood [1]. Autologous HSCT (Auto-HSCT) is transplantation of stem cells, which are collected from the patient by apheresis and stored in a freezer for a while. Before re-transplantation of patients own stem cells, patient should be treated with high-dose chemotherapy (sometimes also with radiotherapy) in order to eradicate malignant cell population in the body. According to the intensity of chemo and radiotherapy to destroy bone marrow, this procedure may be partial or complete myeloablative. After myeloablation, bone marrow

| Leukemias | Lymphoid malignancies | Other diseases |
|---|---|---|
| AML | DLBCL | Acquired SAA |
| ALL | MCL | Acquired AA/PNH |
| CML | FL | Constitutional SAA |
| | | • Fanconi anemia |
| | | • Dyskeratosis congenita |
| Myelofibrosis | WM | Germ cell tumors |
| MDS | TCL | Ewing's sarcoma family of tumors |
| CLL | Primary CTCL | Multiple sclerosis |
| | HL | Systemic scleroderma |
| | MM | Systemic lupus erythematosus |
| | AL | Crohn's disease |
| | | Rheumatoid arthritis |
| | | Vasculitis |
| | | Polymyositis-dermatomyositis |
| | | Cytopenias |

*Note*: AA = aplastic anemia, AML = acute myeloid leukemia, ALL = acute lymphoid leukemia, AL = amyloidosis, CML = chronic myeloid leukemia, CLL = chronic lymphocytic leukemia, CTCL = cutaneous T-cell lymphoma, DLBCL = diffuse large B cell lymphoma, FL = folicular lymphoma, HL = hodgkin lymphoma, MCL = mantle cell lymphoma, MDS = myelodysplastic syndrome, MM = multiple myeloma, PNH = paroxismal nocturnal hemoglobinuria, SAA = severe aplastic anemia, TCL = T-cell lymphoma, WM = waldenstrom macroglobulinemia.

**Table 1.** Indications of HSCT for adults.

is supposed to be free of malignant cells. Patient's own stem cells then reinfused via his/her venous vascular access in order to locate bone marrow and maintain normal hematopoiesis. Patient have the risk of infection during leukopenia, but it is lower in auto- than allo-HSCT because imunosuppression is milder in auto-HSCT. Graft versus host disease (GVHD) is the condition in which white blood cells in the graft (donated blood product) recognize the host as a foreign particle and attack the host's cells. GVHD is so rare but possible in auto-HSCT although the host and the graft are genetically same. Donor in allo-HSCT is another healthy person whose HLA (human leukocyte antigen) type is matched with the recipient. HLA gene complex encodes the major histocompatibility complex (MHC) cell-surface proteins, which regulate immune system. Transplant reactions occur according to the compatibility of HLAs between donor and the recipient. Allogeneic transplant donors can be syngeneic (identical twin), HLA-identical sibling, other family member or unrelated donor (from a volunteer). 10/10 or 8/8 identical donor based on HLA high-resolution typing for class I (HLA-A, -B, -C) and II (HLA-DRB1, -DQB1) is defined as well-matched unrelated donor. A mismatched unrelated donor means that at least one allele at HLA-A, -B, -C or -DR are mismatched [2]. Related donors are relatives or siblings of the patient. Unrelated donors are available by national or

| Hematological malignancies | Non-malignant disorders; solid tumors |
|---|---|
| AML | Primary immunodeficiencies |
| ALL | Thalassemia |
| CML | Sickle cell disease (high risk) |
| NHL | Aplastic anemia |
| HL | Fanconi anemia |
| MDS | Blackfan-Diamond anemia |
| | Chronic granulomatous disease |
| | Kostman's disease |
| | MPS-1H Hurler |
| | MPS-VI Maroteaux-Lamy |
| | Osteopetrosis |
| | Autoimmune diseases |
| | Germ cell tumor |
| | Ewing's sarcoma |
| | Soft tissue sarcoma |
| | Neuroblastoma |
| | Wilm's tumor |
| | Brain tumors |

AML = acute myeloid leukemia, ALL = acute lymphoid leukemia, CML = chronic myeloid leukemia, HL = Hodgkin lymphoma, NHL = non-Hodgkin lymphoma, MDS = myelodysplastic syndrome, MPS = mucopolysaccharidosis.

**Table 2.** Indications of HSCT for children.

international bone marrow donor programs. Syngeneic donor means the monozygotic twin of the patient who is full HLA-matched. Umbilical cord blood is an alternative source for hematopoietic stem cell. It is a kind of allo-HSCT which is usually limited to children and the dose of the infused cells are very low [3]. Because of the similarity between allo-HCST, we will not separately discuss transfusion in umbilical cord blood transplantation.

### 1.2. Indications for HSCT

HSCT is widely performed in hematologic malignancies but also indicated in other solid tumors, and non-malignant diseases. Here are the lists of indications of HSCT for adults and children according to the sixth report from the European Society for Blood and Marrow Transplantation (EBMT) [2] (**Tables 1** and **2**). Because of the wide range of under-investigation indications, we only list diseases for which HSCT is standard of care, generally indicated in suitable patients or clinical option that can be carried after careful assessment of risks and benefits.

## 2. Transfusion in transplantation

HSCT patients need transfusion of blood products before, during and after the transplantation period. As a consequence of increase in the number of HSCTs, need for transfusions increased in the hospitals where transplantations are performed and also other health care centers that are involved in managing these patients. Transfusion in HSCT has unique features such as alloimmunization, ABO-mismatched transplantations, infections and more that will be discussed in detail.

### 2.1. Before transplantation

Recipients of HSCT require special blood components such as leukocyte-reduced, cytomegalovirus (CMV) negative and $\gamma$-irradiated blood components [4, 5].

#### *2.1.1. Leukocyte-reduced erythrocyte and platelet components*

Leukocyte reduction from erythrocyte and platelet products prevents febrile, nonhemolytic transfusion reactions, alloimmunization to HLA antigens and transfusion-transmitted cytomegalovirus (CMV) infections. HLA alloimmunization means formation of antibodies against non-self HLA antigens. Anti-HLA antibodies are inducible by multiple pregnancies and transfusion of blood products (especially if they are not leukocyte-reduced). These antibodies are problematic in HSCT recipient because of the resistance or refractoriness to platelet/erythrocyte transfusion and also cause cross-match positivity against HLA antigens [6]. HLA crossmatch positive allo-HSCT may result with primary graft rejection [6]. Leukocyte reduction filters are not completely effective, some leukocytes and membrane fragments are able to pass through them [5]. In spite of insufficiency to prevent HLA alloimmunization, transfusing only leukocyte-reduced erythrocyte and platelet components to pretransplantation patients is one of the few tools available to potentially reduce the risk of platelet transfusion refractoriness [7].

#### *2.1.2. CMV infection*

CMV serology status of both donor and the recipient is important components of transplantation. CMV transmission from blood products into immunocompromised patients such as transplant recipients can cause fatal infection. Current technologies in prevention of transmission include: provision of CMV-seronegative blood components; postdonation leukocyte reduction filters; and pathogen inactivation, for example, photodynamic therapy with psoralens and UV or visible light [8]. The American Association of Blood Banks states that levels of less than $5 \times 10^6$ leukocytes per blood component may significantly reduce transfusion-transmitted CMV infection [9]. There are also contrary results that support the use of CMV-seronegative products to be superior to leukocyte reduction filters in preventing CMV transmission [10, 11]. The last survey of current practice for prevention of transfusion-transmitted CMV in the United States reported wide variability in the use of leukoreduction versus CMV-seronegative products [12]. CMV serology should be tested for the donor and the recipient. If the recipient is seropositive, the most common CMV infection is reactivation of latent infection; for this reason, using seronegative blood products has little importance. If HSCT is HLA-matched sibling or autologous transplantation, CMV positivity of the patient may be overcome by preemptive antiviral treatment (ganciclovir, foscarnet) with or without high-dose intravenous immunoglobulin [13–15]. CMV infection risk is the highest when CMV seropositive patients receive transplantations from unrelated, HLA-mismatched, or sibling-matched (matched other than genotypic) donors and T lymphocyte-depleted or cord blood allografts [7]. For this reason, most centers routinely administer anti-CMV prophylactic therapy to HSCT recipients in whom immunocompetence is delayed (haploidentical, T-lymphocyte-depleted, and cord blood transplantations) [7]. The risk for CMV infection is so low in seronegative HSCT recipient exposed to only seronegative blood products and CMV negative donor. Obtaining CMV negative blood products is not always easy, and urgent transfusions should not be delayed until seronegative products are available [7].

### 2.1.3. *Transfusion-related graft versus host disease and gamma irradiation*

Transfusion-related graft versus host disease (TR-GVHD) is a complication of blood product transfusion, which contains donor T lymphocytes that engraft in susceptible immunosuppressed host and trigger an immune response against it [16]. TR-GVHD usually develops 4–30 days after the blood transfusion. Viable donor lymphocytes attack recipient's antigen-presenting tissues. The attack is manifested in skin, liver, gastrointestinal tract and bone marrow. Bone marrow involvement distinguishes TR-GVHD from transplantation-related disease. In HSCT, bone marrow is the nest for donor cells so privileged from the attack [17]. Usually donor lymphocytes are destroyed by the recipient's immune system; however, this protection does not work in two conditions: immunodeficiency in the recipient and specific type of partial HLA matching between the donor and the recipient. Examples for immunodeficient states are hematologic cancers, lymphoproliferative disorders, patients with solid tumors and rheumatologic diseases who are immunosuppressed because of chemotherapy or radiotherapy, Congenital immune deficiency, and AIDS [18–20]. Second setting for susceptibility to TR-GVHD is that recipients of blood who are heterozygous for an HLA haplotype for which the donor is homozygous [21]. Donor lymphocytes are not detected as foreign particles by recipient, since the only HLA antigens seen by the host lymphocytes are shared by the recipient. But donor lymphocytes recognize the host's tissues as foreign and initiate an immune attack which is named as TR-GVHD. Blood products associated with TR-GVHD are nonirradiated whole blood, packed red cells, platelets, granulocytes, and fresh and non-frozen plasma. TR-GVHD is not associated with frozen, deglycerolized red cells, fresh frozen plasma, or cryoprecipitate. The early clinical features are fever, maculopapular skin rash, diarrhea and hepatitis occurring 1–2 weeks after transfusion. Later, bone marrow involvement produces severe hypoplasia with profound pancytopenia [22]. Diagnosis is generally made by the biopsy of the affected organs such as skin, gut, and liver, showing evidence of persistence of donor lymphocytes. In order to prove the donor lymphocytes in the host tissue, polymerase chain reaction in peripheral blood [23] or short tandem repeat analysis using peripheral blood and skin biopsies from affected and non-affected sites in the patient, and peripheral blood samples from the implicated donors [24] can be used. The major way for prevention from TR-GVHD is gamma or X-irradiation of blood components, by validated systems. The minimum dose achieved in the irradiation volume should be 25 Gy, not exceeding 50 Gy. Blood components that should be irradiated for at-risk patients are all red cell, platelet, and granulocyte components except cryopreserved red cells after deglycerolization. There is no need to irradiate fresh frozen plasma, cryoprecipitate or fractionated plasma. Also all transfusions from first- or second-degree relatives should be irradiated, even if the patient is immunocompetent. All recipients of allo-HSCT must receive irradiated blood components from the time of initiation of conditioning chemoradiotherapy and should be continued while the patient keeps receiving GVHD prophylaxis. If chronic GVHD exist or immunusupressive treatment is continued, irradiated blood components should be given. Allo-HSCT donors (peripheral blood or bone marrow) should be transfused with irradiated blood 7 days prior to or during the harvest. Auto-HSCT patients should receive irradiated cellular blood components during and for 7 days before the harvest to prevent the collection of viable allogeneic T lymphocytes, which can potentially resist cryopreservation. Otherwise auto-HSCT patients should receive irradiated cellular blood components from initiation of conditioning therapy until 3 months from transplantation (6 months if total body irradiation was used in conditioning) [22].

### 2.2. Peritransplantation

The peritransplantation period begins with immunosuppressive preparation regimen, including stem cell infusion, and until engraftment. HSCT donor must be screened of blood group serology, HLA groups, CMV serology status, donor-recipient size disparity, and donor health. Donor and recipient ABO/Rh (D) types are preferred to be compatible but if not, it does not exclude the HSCT donor volunteering. Nearly one-half of all HSCT involve recipient-donor ABO incompatibility [25].

#### *2.2.1. ABO Incompatibility*

*Major ABO Mismatch*: Donor's erythrocytes are incompatible with recipient's plasma. It occurs most frequently in group O patients who are receiving HSCT from group A, group B, or group AB donors and also when group A and group B recipients receive grafts from group AB donors. Erythrocyte content in the HSC graft should be minimal in order to prevent significant hemolysis after HSCT transfusion. Erythrocytes can be extracted from the donor's bone marrow by Hetastarch separation, mononuclear cell concentration by machine, or through density gradient separation [26]. If a major ABO incompatibility exists, hematocrit should be less than 2% during apheresis collection [7].

*Minor ABO Mismatch*: Donor's plasma is incompatible with recipient's erythrocytes. ABO minor incompatibility may occur in such conditions: (1) if a patient of AB blood group receives HSCT from a non-AB blood group donor, which contains anti-A, anti-B, or both; (2) if a patient from group A receives a B or an O HSCT, which contains anti-A; or (3) if a group B patient receives an A or O transplantation, which contains anti-B [25]. In order to minimize the risk plasma-depleted HSCT products will be collected. The removed plasma volume is proportional to the titer of the offending antibody(s) and the ratio of plasma-to-recipient erythrocyte volume [7].

### 2.2.2. *Transfusion thresholds in peritransplatation period*

Threshold for platelet transfusion is generally 10,000/μL in most transplantation centers [27, 28]. Nevertheless, patient's clinical condition must be the basic determinant for transfusion requirements. Bleeding is common and multifactorial in HSCT patients such as mucositis, hemorrhagic cystitis, GVHD, veno-occlusive disease (VOD), and diffuse alveolar hemorrhage. If the patient has another factor for bleeding, platelet transfusion threshold must be personalised. In HSCT patients, platelet rise may be less efficient than other patient groups as a result of alloimmunization. HLA-matched or crossmatched apheresis platelets are required to overcome alloimmunization.

Hemoglobin threshold for erythrocyte transfusion also varies for different clinical conditions. It can be summarized as follows [29]:

- Hemoglobin < 6 g/dL—transfusion recommended except in exceptional circumstances.
- Hemoglobin 6–7 g/dL—transfusion generally likely to be indicated.
- Hemoglobin 7–8 g/dL—transfusion may be appropriate in patients undergoing orthopedic surgery or cardiac surgery, and also for patients with underlying cardiovascular disease, after evaluation of the patient's clinical needs.
- Hemoglobin 8–10 g/dL—in general, transfusion is not required, but some populations such as patients with symptomatic anemia, with active bleeding, suffering from acute coronary heart disease, and with hematological or oncological malignancies those having thrombocytopenia and at risk of bleeding may need erythrocyte transfusions.
- Hemoglobin > 10 g/dL—transfusion generally not indicated except in exceptional circumstances.

The impact of erythrocyte transfusions on outcome and the hemoglobin threshold in HSCT patients are not well understood. In a recent study, patients with a hematologic malignancy requiring HSCT were randomized to either a restrictive (hemoglobin threshold <7 g/dL) or liberal (hemoglobin threshold < 9 g/dL) erythrocyte transfusion strategies between Day-0 and Day-100. The use of a restrictive red blood cell (RBC) transfusion strategy is compared with a liberal strategy in patients undergoing HSCT as the HRQOL (health-related quality of life) is similar and there are no appreciable differences in HSCT-associated clinical outcomes [30].

### 2.2.3. *Recommendations for ABO/Rh(D) matching*

In HSCT, blood group matching is not required between donor and the recipient, but there are unique transfusion rules that exist. ABO incompatibility is classified as either major, minor, or bidirectional [25] (**Table 3**).

The clinical consequences and management of ABO incompatibilities are discussed below.

| Mismatch type | ABO blood type | | Potential clinical consequence | Etiology | Potential interventions |
|---|---|---|---|---|---|
| | Recipient | Donor | | | |
| Major | 0 | A, B | • Acute hemolysis<br>• Delayed erythrocyte engraftment<br>• Delayed engraftment of granulocyte and Platelets<br>• Pure red blood cell aplasia | • Transfusion of incompatible erythrocytes<br>• Patient anti-donor isohemagglutinins<br>• Loss of immature stem cells from processing<br>• Loss of immature stem cells from processing with ABO antigens expressed on granulocytes and platelets | • Erythrocyte reduction of stem cell product<br>• Therapeutic plasma exchange in recipient to reduce isohemagglutinins before transplantation<br>• Promote donor erythropoiesis via erythropoietin administration |
| | | AB | | | |
| Major | A | AB | | | |
| Major | B | AB | | | |
| Minor | A | O | • Acute hemolysis<br>• Delayed hemolysis secondary to passenger lymphocyte syndrome | • Donor plasma with elevated isohemagglutinin titers/small blood volume recipient<br>• Passenger lymphocytes producingisohemagglutinins | • Plasma reduction<br>• Continual clinical monitoring between days 5 and 15 for signs/symptoms of hemolysis and laboratory monitoring (LDH, bilirubin, complete blood count,DAT) |
| Minor | B | O | | | |
| Minor | AB | O, A, B | | | |
| Bidirectional | A | B | • Combination of major and minor consequences | Combination of major and minor etiologies | Combination of major and minor Bidirectional B A interventions |
| Bidirectional | B | A | | | |

*Note*: LDH = lactate dehydrogenase; DAT = direct antiglobulin test.

**Table 3.** Types of donor-recipient ABO incompatibilities.

### 2.3. After transplantation

ABO-mismatched allo-HSCTs have some complications such as immediate or delayed hemolytic reactions, delayed erythrocyte engraftment and red cell aplasia. Immediate immune hemolysis is usually after HPC transplantation infusion and is due to major ABO mismatch (because of the antibodies in the recipient), whereas delayed hemolysis is a consequence of minor ABO-mismatch (because of donor blood group antibodies) [7]. Several clinical conditions that can mimic immune hemolysis include veno-occlusive disease, GVHD, and thrombotic thrombocytopenic purpura. Direct antiglobulin positivity is highly suspicious for transplant-related immune hemolysis. **Table 4** demonstrates an overview to hemolysis in patients after HSCT [7].

#### *2.3.1. Passenger lymphocyte syndrome*

Passenger lymphocyte syndrome (PLS) occurs when transplanted B lymphocytes produce incompatible blood group antibodies after transplantation [31]. Hemolysis due to PLS may be delayed by 5–15 days after transplantation but is rare after 6–8 weeks [32, 33]. PLS includes ABO incompatibility; additionally, incompatibility in the Rh, Kell, Duffy, or Kidd blood group systems has been reported [34–37]. It is wise to expect higher PLS in peripheral HSCT than bone marrow HSCT because of the higher lymphocyte content in peripheral blood but reports regarding this are mostly anecdotal [7]. Other risk factors for PLS are the use of cyclosporine alone in the absence of an antiproliferative agent, such as methotrexate, for posttransplantation GVHD prophylaxis [38, 32], and the use of a reduced-intensity preparative regimen. After 5–15 days, hemolysis limits itself as the incompatible erythrocytes are eliminated and switched by donor or transfused erythrocytes. "Bystander" immune hemolysis is the term, when hemolysis is more extensive than expected from patient's erythrocytes alone, attributed to hemolysis of transfused compatible erythrocytes [38]. Plasma reduction does not diminish the B lymphocyte content of HSC material and, for this reason, does not affect the incidence of PLS. Rituximab may be used in PLS prevention [39]. Pretransplantation red cell exchange procedures to reduce the volume of donor incompatible erythrocytes in the recipient before infusion are found to be ineffective and associated with a relatively large fraction of residual recipient red cells [40].

The major complications of major ABO-incompatible transplantation include delayed red cell engraftment and pure red cell aplasia (PRCA). Major ABO incompatibilities may cause delay in RBC engraftment. The diagnosis of PRCA is established if reticulocytopenia persists for more than 60 days and erythrocyte precursors are absent in the bone marrow aspirate. In addition, an inverse correlation between ABO hemagglutinin titers and reticulocyte counts exists. In some major ABO incompatible allo-HSCTs, donor hematopoietic stem cells' conversion and RBC production are inhibited by isohemagglutinins produced by recipient plasma [41]. The primary pathology is disruption of normal bone marrow maturation by the recipient isohemagglutinins at the colony-forming-units-ertyhroid stage [42]. Time for recovery of erythropoiesis depends on the pretransplantation titer of antidonor isohemagglutinins, quantity of target antigen available, rate of clearance of isohemagglutinins, presence of GVHD, transplantation-conditioning regimen, and the native recipient erythropoietic function [43, 44]. Resolution of

| Diagnosis | Pathophysiology | Serologic findings |
|---|---|---|
| **HSC graft-related immune hemolysis** | | |
| Major ABO incompatibility between HSC donor and recipient | Hemolysis of transfused erythrocytes, delay in erythrocyte engraftment | DAT positive for C3d, IgG or both; anti-A and/or anti-B present in eluate |
| Minor ABO incompatibility between HSC donor and recipient | Hemolysis of patient's erythrocytes caused by transfused donor's plasma or by passenger lymphocyte-derived isohemagglutinins | DAT positive for C3d, IgG or both anti-A and/or anti-B present in eluate |
| Major incompatibility: other blood group antigens | Hemolysis of transfused donor's erythrocytes | DAT positive for C3d, IgG or both; antibody to non-ABO red blood cell antigen(s) identified in eluate and patient plasma |
| Minor incompatibility: other blood group antigens | Hemolysis of patient's erythrocytes caused by alloantibodies in transfused donor plasma or by passenger lymphocyte-derived alloantibodies | DAT positive for C3d, IgG, or both: antibody to non-ABO red blood cell antigen(s) identified in eluate and patient plasma |
| **Transfusion-related immune hemolysis** | | |
| Transfusion of erythrocytes incompatible with donor or patient | Hemolysis of transfused erythrocytes caused by patient's native or graft-derived antibodies | DAT positive for C3d, IgG or both: anti-A and/or anti-B or antibody to other RBC antigen identified in eluate and patient plasma |
| Transfusion of plasma incompatible with donor or patient | Hemolysis of patient and/or donor erythrocytes | DAT positive for C3d, IgG or both; anti-A and/or anti-B or antibody to other RBC antigen identified in eluate and patient plasma |
| **Other causes of immune hemolysis** | | |
| Autoimmune hemolytic anemia | Hemolysis and serologic incompatibility of (all) crossmatched donor erythrocytes | DAT positive for C3d, IgG or both; panagglutinin present in eluate and patient plasma |
| Drug-induced hemolytic anemia | Autoantibody formation induced by drug, hapten mechanism, or drug modification of erythrocyte membrane | DAT positive for C3d, IgG or both; eluate may react with drug-treated erythrocytes |
| **Nonimmune hemolysis** | | |
| TTP | Microangiopathic hemolytic anemia | DAT and antibody screen negative |
| Cryopreserved stem cell products infusion | Nonimmune hemolysis may be observed during infusion of DMSO-cryopreserved HSC preparations | DAT negative |
| Clostridium perfringens sepsis | C perfringens-produced hemolysin toxins cause nonimmune intravascular hemolysis | DAT negative |

*Note*: HSC = hematopoietic stem cell, DAT = direct antiglobulin test, C3D = complement factor 3D, DMSO = dimethyl sulfoxide, IgG = immunoglobulin G, RBC = red blood cell, TTP = thrombotic thrombocytopenic purpura.

**Table 4.** Differential diagnosis of hemolysis in HSCT patients.

PRA usually takes a few weeks or months but rarely continues for 5 years [45]. Management of PRA includes tapering immunosuppression, using erythropoietin, steroids, plasma exchange, rituximab, and donor lymphocyte infusions [46–48].

### 2.4. Post-engraftment period

There are some clinical conditions specific to post-engraftment of stem cells, which may increase the requirement for blood products.

#### 2.4.1. *Graft-versus host disease*

In acute GVHD cytopenias of 1–3 cell lines and an immune-based hemolytic anemia may occur; also, gastrointestinal GVHD may cause bleeding because of ulcers in gastrointestinal system, and severe liver GVHD may also develop the clotting disturbances [49]. Blood product support during GVHD is essential.

#### 2.4.2. *Hemorrhagic cystitis*

Hemorrhagic cystitis is a toxicity related with cyclophosphamide; however, several viral etiologies, including adenovirus and BK virus, have been reported [50]. HSCT patients with hemorrhagic cystitis may require RBC replacement proportional to its loss and platelet transfusion if the patient is thrombocytopenic. Tranexamic acid should be avoided because of possible clothing within the ureters. Bladder irrigation and platelet transfusion are the mainstay of the treatment.

#### 2.4.3. *Hepatic veno-occlusive disease*

Hepatic veno-occlusive disease (VOD), also known as sinusoidal obstruction syndrome, is a major complication of HSCT and carries a high mortality risk. Many different risk factors for VOD have been described, including platelet transfusions containing ABO-incompatible plasma [51]. Incompatible isoagglutinins to ABO blood-group antigens on hepatic sinusoidal endothelial cells may cause toxic injury initiating a sequence of biological events that may lead to circulatory compromise of centrilobular hepatocytes, fibrosis, and obstruction of blood flow, resulting in VOD [7]. It is wise to think that all platelet transfusions after HSCT should be ABO-compatible with both donor and recipient blood types. In VOD, the need for platelet transfusion is increased as a result of activated coagulation and portal hypertension-related thrombocytopenia.

#### 2.4.4. *Donor lymphocyte infusion*

Donor lymphocyte infusion (DLI) is one of the strategies for managing relapsed hematologic malignancy after HSCT. This procedure is the infusion of lymphocytes from the original stem cell donor after the transplant to augment an antitumor immune response or to be sure that the donor HSCs remain engrafted. Aim is to initiate the process called the graft-versus-tumor effect. T cells of donor are supposed to attack residual cancer cells.

#### 2.4.5. Granulocyte transfusion

Granulocyte transfusion is not routine procedure, but larger doses of granulocytes collection became possible after the discovery and availability of recombinant granulocyte colony-stimulating factor (G-CSF) increased the interest for the issue [52]. It is possible to collect $5–10 \times 10^{10}$ granulocytes at once [53–55]. Some authors recommend granulocyte transfusion in patients meet that criterion regardless of the cause of neutropenia [56]:

- Absolute neutrophil count <500 cells/μL, except in the case of chronic granulomatous disease.
- Evidence of bacterial or fungal infection (i.e., clinical symptoms of infection, positive cultures, pathological diagnosis of infection from biopsies, radiographic evidence of pneumonia).
- Unresponsiveness to antimicrobial treatment for at least 48 hours (except in extreme circumstances with life-threatening infection)

Chemotherapy and HSCT are the most common indications for granulocyte transfusion even though their use is rare in daily practice. Family members and community donors both can donate granulocytes; however, donor must fulfill some criterion. Donors must be ABO and Rh-matched to the recipient, negative for all blood transfusion-associated infectious disease markers within 30 days of granulocyte donation, having good vascular access, and not be pregnant and having hemoglobinopathy. G-CSF (300 mcg subcutaneously) and dexamethasone (8 mg orally) are administered on the day prior to each collection [54]. Granulocyte harvesting by apheresis is performed by removing granulocytes and returning erythrocytes and plasma to the donor. Adverse reactions associated with granulocyte transfusion are pulmonary adverse reactions [57], transfusion-associated GVHD [58], alloimmunization [59], and infections [60], especially CMV [61].

#### 2.4.6. Erythrocyte chimerism

Allo-HSCT patients should be assessed with chimerism studies in order to detect the genotypic origin of posttransplant hematopoiesis. This study serves to define engraftment, graft failure, and relapse. Complete chimerism means hematopoiesis is entirely from the donor; mixed chimerism is the condition that a variable ratio of donor- to recipient-derived cells, and engraftment failure means cells are all from the recipient. Blood group chimerism is an important issue in allo-HSCT patients. According to ABO matching, varied incidences of ABO-grouping discrepancies or mixed field-agglutination reactions have been reported [7]. Antierythrocyte antibodies are measured to document erythrocyte chimerism, once the patient's blood becomes full-donor chimera, recipient-derived antierythrocyte antibodies disappear. Then, blood products consistent with donor ABO typing should be used. After establishing full donor engraftment, the onset of mixed erythrocyte chimerism (circulating erythrocytes typing with mixed field-donor recipient ABO groups) may be signaling for the relapse and/or graft failure [62].

Transfusion-support recommendations for ABO incompatible HSCT are summarized in **Table 5** [25].

http://dx.doi.org/10.5772/intechopen.69260

| Recipient | Donor | Phase 1 | Phase 2 | | | | | Phase 3 | | | | |
|---|---|---|---|---|---|---|---|---|---|---|---|---|
| | | All products | RBC's | Platelets | | Plasma | | RBC's | Platelets | | Plasma | |
| | | | | 1st Choice | 2nd Choices | 1st Choice | 2nd Choices | | 1st Choice | 2nd Choices | 1st Choice | 2nd Choices |
| O | A | Recipient | O | A | AB, B, O | A | AB | Donor | A | AB, B, O | A | AB |
| O | B | Recipient | O | B | AB, A, O | B | AB | Donor | B | AB, A, O | B | AB |
| O | AB | Recipient | O | AB | A, B, O | AB | NA | Donor | AB | A, B, O | AB | NA |
| A | AB | Recipient | A | AB | A, B, O | AB | NA | Donor | AB | A, B, O | AB | NA |
| B | AB | Recipient | B | AB | B, A, O | AB | NA | Donor | AB | B, A, O | AB | NA |
| A | O | Recipient | O | A | AB, B, O | A | AB | Donor | A | AB, B, O | A | AB |
| B | O | Recipient | O | B | AB, A, O | B | AB | Donor | B | AB, A, O | B | AB |
| AB | O | Recipient | O | AB | A, B, O | AB | NA | Donor | AB | A, B, O | AB | NA |
| AB | A | Recipient | A | AB | A, B, O | AB | NA | Donor | AB | A, B, O | AB | NA |
| AB | B | Recipient | B | AB | B, A, O | AB | NA | Donor | AB | B, A, O | AB | NA |
| A | B | Recipient | O | AB | B, A, O | AB | NA | Donor | AB | B, A, O | AB | NA |
| B | A | Recipient | O | AB | O, A, B | AB | NA | Donor | AB | A, B, O | AB | NA |

*Note*: NA = not applicable; Phase 1 = time period between diagnosis and transplantation; Phase 2 = time period between transplantation and RBC engraftment; Phase 3 = engraftment established, as indicated by direct antiglobulin testing being negative, along with two consecutive separate samples with the forward and reverse typing showing donor ABO status.

**Table 5.** Transfusion support recommendations for ABO incompatible HSCT.

Autologous and allogeneic HSCT are associated with pancytopenia in the pre-, peri-, and posttransplant period. Blood product transfusion is an inevitable and critical component for the patient management. HSCT patients have special requirements regarding blood products transfusion. Transfusion services, hospitals, physicians, and other health care staff who take care of transplant patients should be aware of that those patients have specific and specialized transfusion requirements.

## Author details

Eren Arslan Davulcu, Fahri Sahin and Güray Saydam*

*Address all correspondence to: saydamguray@yahoo.com

Hematology Department, Faculty of Medicine, Ege University, Bornova, İzmir, Turkey

## References

[1] Copelan EA. Hematopoietic stem-cell transplantation. The New England Journal of Medicine. 2006;**354**:1813-1826

[2] Sureda A, Bader P, Cesaro S, Dreger P, Duarte RF, et al. Indications for allo- and auto-SCT for haematological diseases, solid tumours and immune disorders: Current practice in Europe, 2015. Bone Marrow Transplantation. 2015;**50**:1037-1056

[3] Ballen KK, Gluckman E, Broxmeyer HE. Umbilical cord blood transplantation: The first 25 years and beyond. Blood. 2013; **122**(4):491-498

[4] Klumpp TR. Immunohematologic complications of bone marrow transplantation. Bone Marrow Transplantation. 1991;**8**:159-170

[5] The Trial to Reduce Alloimmunization to Platelets Study Group. Leukocyte reduction and ultraviolet B irradiation of platelets to prevent alloimmunization and refractoriness to platelet transfusions. The New England Journal of Medicine. 1997;**337**:1861-1869

[6] Kaminski ER, Hows JM, Goldman JM, Batchelor JR. Pretransfused patients with severe aplastic anaemia exhibit high numbers of cytotoxic T lymphocyte precursors probably directed at non-HLA antigens. British Journal of Haematology. 1990;**76**:401-405

[7] Gajewski JL, Johnson VV, Sandler SG, Sayegh A, Klumpp TR. A review of transfusion practice before, during, and after hematopoietic progenitor cell transplantation. Blood. 2008; **112**(8):3036-3047

[8] Radia R, Pamphilon D. Transfusion strategies in patients undergoing stem-cell transplantation. Expert Review of Hematology. 2011;**4**(2):213-220

[9] American Association of Blood Banks. Technical Manual. 15th ed. Bethesda, MD: American Association of Blood Banks; 2005.

[10] Nichols WG, Price TH, Gooley T, Corey L, Boeckh M. Transfusion-transmitted cytomegalovirus infection after receipt of leuko-reduced blood products. Blood. 2003;**101**:4195-4200

[11] Vamvakas EC. Is white blood cell reduction equivalent to antibody screening in preventing transmission of cytomegalovirus by transfusion? A review of the literature and meta-analysis. Transfusion Medicine Reviews. 2005;**19**(3):181-199

[12] Smith D, Lu Q, Yuan S, Goldfinger D, Fernando LP, Ziman A. Survey of current practice for prevention of transfusion transmitted cytomegalovirus in the United States: Leucoreduction vs cytomegalovirus seronegative. Vox Sanguinis. 2010;**98**(1):29-36

[13] Winston DJ, Ho WG, Bartoni K, et al. Ganciclovir prophylaxis of cytomegalovirus infection and disease in allogeneic bone marrow transplant recipients: Results of a placebo-controlled, double-blind trial. Annals of Internal Medicine. 1993;**118**:179-184

[14] Fraser GAM, Walker II. Canadian Blood and Marrow Transplant Group. Cytomegalovirus prophylaxis and treatment after hematopoietic stem cell transplantation in Canada: A description of current practices and comparison with Centers for Disease Control/Infectious Diseases Society of America/America Society for Blood and Marrow Transplantation guideline recommendations. Biology of Blood and Marrow Transplantation. 2004;**10**:287-297

[15] Bass EB, Powe NR, Goodman SN, et al. Efficacy of immune globulin in preventing complications of bone marrow transplantation: A meta-analysis. Bone Marrow Transplantation. 1993;**12**:273-282

[16] Petz LD, Calhoun L, Yam P, et al. Transfusionassociated graft-versus-host disease in immunocompetent patients: Report of a fatal case associated with transfusion of blood from a second degree relative, and a survey of predisposing factors. Transfusion. 1993;**33**:742-750

[17] Ferrara JL, Deeg HJ. Graft-versus-host disease. The New England Journal of Medicine. 1991; **324**(10):667

[18] Schroeder ML. Transfusion-associated graft-versus-host disease. British Journal of Haematology. 2002;**117**(2):275

[19] Maung ZT, Wood AC, Jackson GH, Turner GE, Appleton AL, Hamilton PJ. Transfusion-associated graft-versus-host disease in fludarabine-treated B-chronic lymphocytic leukaemia. British Journal of Haematology. 1994;**88**(3):649

[20] Leitman SF, Tisdale JF, Bolan CD, Popovsky MA, Klippel JH, Balow JE, Boumpas DT, Illei GG. Transfusion-associated GVHD after fludarabine therapy in a patient with systemic lupus erythematosus. Transfusion. 2003;**43**(12):1667

[21] Shivdasani RA, Haluska FG, Dock NL, Dover JS, Kineke EJ, Anderson KC. Brief report: Graft-versus-host disease associated with transfusion of blood from unrelated HLA-homozygous donors. The New England Journal of Medicine. 1993;**328**(11):766

[22] Treleaven J, Gennery A, Marsh J, Norfolk D, Page L, Parker A, Saran F, Thurston J, Webb D. Guidelines on the use of irradiated blood components prepared by the British Committee for Standards in Haematology blood transfusion task force. British Journal of Haematology. 2011;**152**(1):35-51

[23] Utter GH, Reed WF, Lee TH, Busch MP. Transfusion associated microchimerism. Vox Sanguinis. 2007;**93**:188-195. DOI: 10.1111/j.1423-0410.2007.00954

[24] Sage D, Stanworth S, Turner D, Navarrete C. Diagnosis of transfusion associated graft-vs.-host disease: The importance of short tandem repeat analysis. Transfusion Medicine. 2005;**15**:481-485

[25] Booth GS, Gehrie EA, Bolan CD, Savani BN. Clinical guide to ABO-incompatible allogeneic stem cell transplantation. Biology of Blood and Marrow Transplantation. 2013;**19**(8): 1152-1158

[26] Braine HG, Sensenrenner LL, Wright SK, Tutschka PJ, Saral R, Santos GW. Bone marrow transplantation with major ABO blood group incompatibility using erythrocyte depletion of marrow before infusion. Blood. 1982;**60**:420-425

[27] Diedrich B, Remberger M, Shanwell A, Svahn BM, Ringden O. A prospective randomized trial of a prophylactic platelet transfusion trigger of $10 \times 10^9$/L versus $30 \times 10^9$/L in allogeneic hematopoietic progenitor cell transplant recipients. Transfusion. 2005;**45**:1064-1072

[28] Nevo S, Fuller AK, Hartley E, Borinsky ME,Vogelsang GB. Acute bleeding complications in patients after hematopoietic stem cell transplantation with prophylactic platelet transfusion triggers of $10 \times 10^9$ and $20 \times 10^9$/L. Transfusion. 2007;**47**:801-812

[29] Carson JL, Guyatt G, Heddle NM, Grossman BJ, Cohn CS, Fung MK, Gernsheimer T, Holcomb JB, Kaplan LJ, Katz LM, Peterson N, Ramsey G, Rao SV, Roback JD, Shander A, Tobian AA. Clinical practice guidelines from the AABB: Red blood cell transfusion thresholds and storage. The Journal of the American Medical Association. 2016;**316**(19):2025

[30] Tay J, Allan DS, Chatelain E, Coyle D, Elemary M, et al. Transfusion of red cells in hematopoietic stem cell transplantation (TRIST Study): A randomized controlled trial evaluating 2 red cell transfusion thresholds. Blood. 2016;**128**:1032

[31] Daniel-Johnson J, Schwartz J. How do I approach ABO-incompatible hematopoietic progenitor cell transplantation? Transfusion. 2011;**51**:1143-1149

[32] Hows J, Beddow K, Gordon-Smith E, et al. Donor-derived red blood cell antibodies and immune hemolysis after allogeneic bone marrow transplantation. Blood. 1986;**67**:177-181

[33] Lee JH, Gulbis A, De Padua Silva L, et al. Rituximab for passenger lymphocyte syndrome associated with allogeneic SCT. Bone Marrow Transplantation. 2008;**42**:67-69

[34] Worel N, Greinix HT, Keil F, et al. Severe immune hemolysis after minor ABO-mismatched allogeneic peripheral blood progenitor cell transplantation occurs more frequently after nonmyeloablative than myeloablative conditioning. Transfusion. 2002;**42**:1293-1301

[35] Zupanska B, Zaucha JM, Michalewska B, Malinowska A, Brojer E, Hellman Al. Multiple red cell alloantibodies, including anti-Dib, after allogeneic ABO-matched peripheral blood progenitor cell transplantation. Transfusion. 2005;**45**:16-20

[36] Cid J, Lozano M, Fernandez-Aviles F, et al. Anti-D alloimmunization after D-mismatched allogeneic hematopoietic stem cell transplantation in patients with hematologic diseases. Transfusion. 2006;**46**:169-173

[37] Leo A, Mytilineos J, Voso MT, et al. Passenger lymphocyte syndrome with severe hemolytic anemia due to an anti-Jk(a) after allogeneic PBPC transplantation. Transfusion. 2000;**40**: 632-636

[38] Gajewski JL, Petz LD, Calhoun L, et al. Hemolysis of transfused group O red blood cells in minor ABO-incompatible unrelated-donor bone marrow transplants in patients receiving cyclosporine without posttransplant methotrexate. Blood. 1992;**79**:3076-3085

[39] Yazer MH, Triulzi DJ. Immune hemolysis following ABO-mismatched stem cell or solid organ transplantation. Current Opinion in Hematology. 2007;**14**:664-670

[40] Worel N, Greinix HT, Supper V, et al. Prophylactic red blood cell exchange for prevention of severe immune hemolysis in minor ABO-mismatched allogeneic peripheral blood progenitor cell transplantation after reduced-intensity conditioning. Transfusion. 2007;**47**:1494-1502

[41] Griffith LM, McCoy JP, Bolan CD, et al. Persistence of recipient plasma cells and anti donor isohemagglutinins in patients with delayed donor erythropoiesis after major ABO incompatible nonmyeloablative haematopietic cell transplantation. British Journal of Haematology. 2005;**128**:668-675

[42] Barge AJ, Johnson G, Witherspoon R, Torok-Storb B. Antibody-mediated marrow failure after allogeneic bone marrow transplantation. Blood. 1989;**74**:1477-1480

[43] Giralt S, Estey E, Albitar M, et al. Engraftment of allogeneic hematopoietic progenitor cells with purine analog-containing chemotherapy: Harnessing graft-versus-leukemia without myeloablative therapy. Blood. 1997;**89**:4531-4536

[44] Bardos A, Tricot G, Toor A, et al. ABO mismatch may affect engraftment in multiple myeloma patients receiving nonmyeloablative conditioning. Transfusion. 2002;**45**:205-209

[45] Volin L, Ruutu T. Pure red-cell aplasia of long duration after major ABO incompatible bone marrow transplantation. Acta Haematologica. 1990;**84**:195-197

[46] Taniguchi S, Yamasaki K, Shibuya T, et al. Recombinant human erythropoietin for long term persistent anemia after major ABO incompatible bone marrow transplantation. Bone Marrow Transplantation. 1993;**12**:423

[47] Bavaro P, Di Girolamo G, Olioso P, et al. Donor lymphocyte infusion as therapy for pure red cell aplasia following bone marrow transplantation. British Journal of Haematology. 1999;**104**:930-931

[48] Sorà F, De Matteis S, Piccirillo N, et al. Rituximab for pure red cell aplasia after ABO-mismatched allogeneic peripheral blood progenitor cell transplantation. Transfusion. 2005;**45**:643-645

[49] Pihusch M. Bleeding complications after hematopoietic stem cell transplantation. Seminars in Hematology. 2004;**41**(Suppl 1):93-100

[50] Seber A, Shu XO, Defor T, Sencer S, Ramsay N. Risk factors for severe hemorrhagic cystitis following BMT. Bone Marrow Transplantation. 1999;**23**:35-40

[51] Lapierre V, Mahé C, Aupérin A, Stambouli F, Oubouzar N, Tramalloni D, Benhamou E, Tiberghien P, Hartmann O. Platelet transfusion containing ABO-incompatible plasma and hepatic veno-occlusive disease after hematopoietic transplantation in young children. Transplantation. 2005;**80**:314-319

[52] Hübel K, Dale DC, Engert A, Liles WC. Current status of granulocyte (neutrophil) transfusion therapy for infectious diseases. The Journal of Infectious Diseases. 2001;**183**(2):321

[53] Liles WC, Huang JE, Llewellyn C, SenGupta D, Price TH, Dale DC. A comparative trial of granulocyte-colony-stimulating factor and dexamethasone, separately and in combination, for the mobilization of neutrophils in the peripheral blood of normal volunteers. Transfusion. 1997;**37**(2):182

[54] Dale DC, Liles WC, Llewellyn C, Rodger E, Price TH. Neutrophil transfusions: Kinetics and functions of neutrophils mobilized with granulocyte-colony-stimulating factor and dexamethasone. Transfusion. 1998;**38**(8):713

[55] Stroncek DF, Yau YY, Oblitas J, Leitman SF. Administration of G--CSF plus dexamethasone produces greater granulocyte concentrate yields while causing no more donor toxicity than G--CSF alone. Transfusion. 2001;**41**(8):1037

[56] Bishton M, Chopra R. The role of granulocyte transfusions in neutropenic patients. British Journal of Haematology. 2004;**127**(5):501

[57] Hester JP, Dignani MC, Anaissie EJ, Kantarjian HM, O'Brien S, Freireich EJ. Collection and transfusion of granulocyte concentrates from donors primed with granulocyte stimulating factor and response of myelosuppressed patients with established infection. Journal of Clinical Apheresis. 1995;**10**(4):188

[58] Capon SM, DePond WD, Tyan DB, Pepkowitz SH, Toyoda H, Cinman AC, Azer PC, Goldfinger D. Transfusion-associated graft-versus-host disease in an immunocompetent patient. Annals of Internal Medicine. 1991;**114**(12):1025

[59] O'Donghaile D, Childs RW, Leitman SF. Blood consult: Granulocyte transfusions to treat invasive aspergillosis in a patient with severe aplastic anemia awaiting mismatched hematopoietic progenitor cell transplantation. Blood. 2012;**119**(6):1353

[60] Schreiber GB, Busch MP, Kleinman SH, Korelitz JJ. The risk of transfusion-transmitted viral infections. The Retrovirus Epidemiology Donor Study. The New England Journal of Medicine. 1996;**334**(26):1685

[61] Nichols WG, Price T, Boeckh M. Cytomegalovirus infections in cancer patients receiving granulocyte transfusions. Blood. 2002;**99**(9):3483

[62] Khan F, Agarwal A, Agrawal S. Significance of chimerism in hematopoietic stem cell transplantation: new variations on an old theme. Bone Marrow Transplantation. 2004;**34**:1-12

# Chapter 7

# Red Blood Cell Transfusion Strategy for Upper Gastrointestinal Bleeding

Xingshun Qi, Fernando Gomes Romeiro and
Yiling Li

Additional information is available at the end of the chapter

http://dx.doi.org/10.5772/intechopen.68804

**Abstract**

Acute upper gastrointestinal bleeding (UGIB) is a potentially lethal and frequent digestive disease. It is mainly divided into the nonvariceal UGIB and variceal bleeding according to the source of bleeding. Red blood cell transfusion is the core therapeutic option for the management of acute UGIB. In this chapter, we reviewed the primary evidence from meta-analyses and large-scale randomized controlled trials regarding red blood cell transfusion strategy for acute UGIB.

**Keywords:** red blood cell, transfusion, upper gastrointestinal bleeding, variceal bleeding, peptic ulcer, management, hemoglobin

## 1. Introduction: Upper gastrointestinal bleeding

### 1.1. Definition

Traditionally, gastrointestinal bleeding is divided into upper and lower gastrointestinal bleeding according to the site of gastrointestinal tract. Upper gastrointestinal bleeding (UGIB) refers to the occurrence of bleeding above the ligament of Treitz, which is often characterized by hematemesis and/or melena; by contrast, lower gastrointestinal bleeding refers to the occurrence of bleeding below the ligament of Treitz. Currently, some researchers also propose the term "mid gastrointestinal bleeding," which refers to the occurrence of bleeding between the ligament of Treitz and ileocecal valve.

### 1.2. Incidence

UGIB is one of the most common emergency diseases. The epidemiological data are heterogeneous among regions. In the UK, an audit study identified a total 6750 patients with acute UGIB from 208 hospitals during a 2-month period (May 1–June 30, 2007) [1]. In Wales, there were 22,299 patients with 24,421 admissions for UGIB during an 8-year period (1999–2007) [2]. The hospitalized incidence of UGIB was estimated to be 134 per 100,000 [2]. In Iceland, a prospective population-based study involving 1731 patients undergoing 2058 upper gastrointestinal endoscopies demonstrated that the annual incidence of acute UGIB was 87/100,000 inhabitants [3]. The data were also heterogeneous among periods. In Italy, there were 532 patients with 587 admissions during a 2-year period from 1983 to 1985 and 513 patients with 539 admissions during a 2-year period from 2002 to 2004 [4]. In Crete, Greece, a population-based study found that the annual incidence of acute UGIB was 160/100,000 during a 1-year period from 1998 to 1999 and 95/100,000 during a 1-year period from 2008 to 2009 [5]. In Achaia, Greece, a population-based study found that the annual incidence of acute UGIB was 162.9/100,000 and 108.3/100,000 in1995 and 2005, respectively [6].

### 1.3. Mortality

UGIB is a potentially lethal disease. Until now, there are lots of data regarding the mortality of patients with UGIB. The mortality is about 10% [1, 2, 7]. A majority of evidence suggests that the mortality is being decreased with time. Loperfido et al. reported that the annual mortality of UGIB decreased from 17.1/100,000 during the period of 1983–1985 to 8.2/100,000 during the period of 2002–2004 [4]. Paspatis et al. also reported that the annual mortality of UGIB decreased from 9/100,000 during the period of 1998–1999 to 6.3/100,000 during the period of 2008–2009 [5]. However, Theocharis et al. found that the overall mortality increased from 3.9% in 1995 to 6.5% in 2005, but no statistically significant difference was found between the two periods [6].

### 1.4. Causes

Peptic ulcer, which primarily refers to gastric and duodenal ulcer, and gastroesophageal varices, which is primarily caused by liver cirrhosis, are the two most common causes of UGIB [8, 9]. First, the major risk factors of peptic ulcer are recent use of nonsteroidal anti-inflammatory drugs (NSAIDs) and anti-platelet agents, *Helicobacter pylori* infection, Zollinger-Ellison syndrome, and smoking [8, 9]. Aspirin is the most widely used NSAID associated with the development of peptic ulcer, especially in patients with previous history of cardiovascular or cerebrovascular diseases. Second, the major etiologies of gastroesophageal varices include liver cirrhosis, portal vein obstruction, and Budd-Chiari syndrome.

Additional causes of UGIB include malignancy, Mallory-Weiss tears, acute inflammation and erosion of esophageal, gastric, and duodenal mucosa, Dieulafoy's lesions, gastric antral vascular ectasia, and arteriovenous malformations.

## 2. Current treatment strategy of UGIB

UGIB is often divided into nonvariceal UGIB and variceal bleeding, because the treatment strategy is greatly different between them.

### 2.1. Nonvariceal UGIB

Several high-impact consensus and practice guidelines have clearly established the recommendations regarding the management of nonvariceal UGIB. First, in the International Consensus UGIB (ICON-UGIB) conference, the management strategy mainly includes five major sections, as follows: (1) resuscitation, risk assessment, and pre-endoscopy management; (2) endoscopic management; (3) pharmacologic management; (4) nonendoscopic and nonpharmacologic in-hospital management; and (5) post-discharge, acetylsalicylic acid, and NSAIDs [10]. Second, the Asia-Pacific Working Group proposes the consensus statements regarding the management of nonvariceal UGIB as follows: pre-endoscopy prognostic scale, early discharge, use of proton pump inhibitor, timing of endoscopic intervention, endoscopic treatment plus proton pump inhibitor, necessity of second-look endoscopy, angiographic embolization, and use of NSAIDs, aspirin, and/or clopidogrel in specific population [11]. Third, the European Society of Gastrointestinal Endoscopy (ESGE) guideline makes the main recommendations in the following parts: (1) initial patient evaluation and hemodynamic resuscitation; (2) risk stratification; (3) pre-endoscopy management; (4) endoscopic therapy; and (5) post-endoscopy/endoscopic hemostasis management [12].

### 2.2. Variceal bleeding

Recently, the recommendations regarding the management of variceal bleeding are primarily obtained from the UK practice guideline [13], Baveno VI consensus [14], American Association for the Study of Liver Diseases (AASLD) practice guidance [15], and the Standards of Practice Committee of the American Society for Gastrointestinal Endoscopy (ASGE) [16]. In general, the main management strategy is classified as follows: (1) screening for varices; (2) primary prophylaxis of variceal bleeding; (3) treatment of acute variceal bleeding; and (4) secondary prophylaxis of variceal bleeding.

## 3. Red blood cell transfusion for acute UGIB

### 3.1. Recommendations from practice guideline and consensus

In nearly all practice guidelines and consensus, a restrictive red blood cell transfusion strategy is proposed.

As for nonvariceal UGIB, the ICON-UGIB recommends that the threshold of initiating red blood cell transfusion should be a hemoglobin level of ≤70 g/L, but does not establish a target of red blood cell transfusion [10]; the ESGE guideline recommends that the target of red blood cell transfusion should be a hemoglobin level of 70–90 g/L in general population and should be moderately elevated in specific population, such as ischemic cardiovascular diseases [12].

As for variceal bleeding, the UK practice guideline recommends that the target of red blood cell transfusion should be a hemoglobin level of 70–80 g/L in hemodynamically stable patients [13]; the Baveno VI consensus recommends that the target of packed red blood cell transfusion should be a hemoglobin level of 70–80 g/L and should be modified according to the cardiovascular disorders, age, hemodynamic status, and ongoing bleeding [14]; the AASLD practice guidance recommends that the threshold of initiating packed red blood cell transfusion should be a hemoglobin level of ≤70 g/L, and the target should be a hemoglobin level of 70–90 g/L [15].

### 3.2. Evidence from meta-analyses

Several meta-analyses have been published regarding red blood cell transfusion for the management of UGIB. First, in 2009, Hearnshaw et al. did a Cochrane systematic review and meta-analysis of three trials including 126 patients [17]. The authors suggested no sufficient data regarding the outcomes of red blood cell transfusion for the management of UGIB. Second, in 2010, Jairath et al. updated the Cochrane systematic review [18]. However, no new data were found. The conclusions were unchanged. In 2013, our team did a meta-analysis of four studies and found that restrictive red blood cell transfusion was superior to liberal red blood cell transfusion for the improvement of overall survival, but the risk of rebleeding was similar between the two red blood cell transfusion strategies [19]. However, it should be noted that the characteristics and definitions of restrictive transfusion were heterogeneous among the included studies.

### 3.3. Evidence from major individual studies

There were two large-scale randomized controlled trials comparing the efficacy and safety of restrictive versus liberal red blood cell transfusion for acute UGIB.

A Spanish, single-center, randomized controlled trial enrolled 921 patients with acute UGIB between 2003 and 2009, in which 461 and 460 patients were assigned to restrictive and liberal red blood cell transfusion groups, respectively [20]. In the restrictive transfusion group, the threshold of initiating red blood cell transfusion was a hemoglobin level of ≤70 g/L, and the target was a hemoglobin level of 70–90 g/L. In the liberal red blood cell transfusion group, the threshold of initiating red blood cell transfusion was a hemoglobin level of ≤90 g/L, and the target was a hemoglobin level of 90–110 g/L. First, the most remarkable finding was that restrictive red blood cell transfusion could significantly decrease the incidence of 6-week death in the overall analysis (5% [23/444] versus 9% [41/445], $P = 0.02$, hazard ratio = 0.55, 95% confidence interval = 0.33–0.92). However, restrictive red blood cell transfusion could not significantly influence the incidence of 6-week death in the subgroup analyses of patients with bleeding from varices (11% [11/93] versus 18% [17/97], $P = 0.18$, hazard ratio = 0.58, 95% confidence interval = 0.27–1.27) or peptic ulcer (3% [7/228] versus 5% [11/209], $P = 0.26$, hazard ratio = 0.70, 95% confidence interval = 0.26–1.25). Second, restrictive red blood cell transfusion could significantly decrease the incidence of further bleeding in the overall analysis (10% [45/444] versus 16% [71/445], $P = 0.01$, hazard ratio = 0.62, 95% confidence interval = 0.43–0.91). However, restrictive red blood cell transfusion could not significantly influence the incidence of further bleeding in the subgroup analyses of patients with bleeding from varices (11% [10/93] versus 22% [21/97], $P = 0.05$, hazard ratio = 0.50, 95% confidence interval = 0.23–0.99) or peptic ulcer (10% [23/228] versus 16% [33/209], $P = 0.09$, hazard ratio = 0.63, 95% confidence interval = 0.37–1.07).

A UK multi-center pragmatic, open-label, cluster randomized trial enrolled 936 patients with acute UGIB between 2012 and 2013, in which 403 and 533 patients were assigned to restrictive and liberal red blood cell transfusion groups, respectively [21]. In the restrictive transfusion group, the threshold of initiating red blood cell transfusion was a hemoglobin level of ≤80 g/L, and the target was a hemoglobin level of 80–100 g/L. In the liberal red blood cell transfusion group, the threshold of initiating red blood cell transfusion was a hemoglobin level of ≤100 g/L, and the target was a hemoglobin level of 100–120 g/L. Neither 28-day mortality (5% [14/257] versus 7% [25/383]) nor further bleeding (5% [13/257] versus 9% [31/383]) was significantly decreased by the restrictive transfusion strategy. No subgroup analyses according to the source of bleeding were available.

### 3.4. Real-world practice

Despite the restrictive red blood cell transfusion strategy is clearly recommended by the major practice guidelines and consensus, not all clinicians fulfilled this policy in clinical practice. A UK survey of six clinical scenarios regarding red blood cell transfusion triggers for acute UGIB in different clinical conditions was conducted in 815 clinicians [22]. A majority of clinicians would like to choose a red blood cell transfusion trigger of 60–100 g/L, and only a minority of clinicians agreed to choose a red blood cell transfusion trigger of ≥100 g/L. Compared with the surgeons, the physicians preferred to choose a higher red blood cell transfusion trigger. A Canadian survey of seven clinical vignettes regarding red blood cell transfusion threshold for acute UGIB in different clinical conditions was conducted in 203 clinicians [23]. The red blood cell transfusion threshold was a mean hemoglobin level of 71 and 86.7 g/L in hemodynamically stable and unstable patients, respectively; a mean hemoglobin level of 84, 74.4, and 71 g/L in patients with coronary artery disease, with liver cirrhosis, and without previous disease history, respectively.

## 4. Conclusions

Acute UGIB is a lethal and frequent digestive disease. A restrictive red blood cell transfusion has been clearly recommended by the practice guidelines and consensus. Generally, the threshold for initiating red blood cell transfusion should be often a hemoglobin level of ≤70 g/L, and the target of red blood cell transfusion should be a hemoglobin level of 70–80 or 70–90 g/L (**Table 1**). However, based on two large-scale randomized controlled trials, we could

| Guideline or consensus | Nonvariceal UGIB | Variceal UGIB |
|---|---|---|
| International Consensus UGIB (ICON-UGIB) | Hemoglobin ≤ 70 g/L | |
| European Society of Gastrointestinal Endoscopy (ESGE) | Hemoglobin 70–90 g/L | |
| United Kingdom practice guideline | | Hemoglobin 70–80 g/L |
| Baveno VI consensus | | Hemoglobin 70–80 g/L |
| American Association for the Study of Liver Diseases practice guidance | | Hemoglobin ≤ 70 g/L |

**Table 1.** Current recommendations from guideline and consensus regarding red blood cell transfusion.

not establish any strong recommendations regarding restrictive red blood cell transfusion in individual patients with variceal bleeding or nonvariceal UGIB. Additionally, in clinical practice, not all clinicians completely fulfilled a restrictive red blood cell transfusion strategy.

## Author details

Xingshun Qi[1]*, Fernando Gomes Romeiro[2] and Yiling Li[3]

*Address all correspondence to: xingshunqi@126.com

1 Department of Gastroenterology, General Hospital of Shenyang Military Area, Shenyang, China

2 Department of Internal Medicine, Botucatu Medical School, Universidade Estadual Paulista (UNESP), Botucatu, SP, Brazil

3 Department of Gastroenterology, First Affiliated Hospital of China Medical University, Shenyang, China

## References

[1] Hearnshaw SA, Logan RF, Lowe D, Travis SP, Murphy MF, Palmer KR. Acute upper gastrointestinal bleeding in the UK: Patient characteristics, diagnoses and outcomes in the 2007 UK audit. Gut. 2011;**60**:1327-1335

[2] Button LA, Roberts SE, Evans PA, Goldacre MJ, Akbari A, Dsilva R, et al. Hospitalized incidence and case fatality for upper gastrointestinal bleeding from 1999 to 2007: A record linkage study. Alimentary Pharmacology & Therapeutics. 2011;**33**:64-76

[3] Hreinsson JP, Kalaitzakis E, Gudmundsson S, Bjornsson ES. Upper gastrointestinal bleeding: incidence, etiology and outcomes in a population-based setting. Scandinavian Journal of Gastroenterology. 2013;**48**:439-447

[4] Loperfido S, Baldo V, Piovesana E, Bellina L, Rossi K, Groppo M, et al. Changing trends in acute upper-GI bleeding: A population-based study. Gastrointestinal Endoscopy. 2009;**70**:212-224

[5] Paspatis GA, Konstantinidis K, Chalkiadakis I, Tribonias G, Chlouverakis G, Roussomoustakaki M. Changing trends in acute upper gastrointestinal bleeding in Crete, Greece: A population-based study. European Journal of Gastroenterology & Hepatology. 2012;**24**:102-103

[6] Theocharis GJ, Thomopoulos KC, Sakellaropoulos G, Katsakoulis E, Nikolopoulou V. Changing trends in the epidemiology and clinical outcome of acute upper gastrointestinal bleeding in a defined geographical area in Greece. Journal of Clinical Gasroenterology. 2008;**42**:128-133

[7] Katschinski BD, Logan RF, Davies J, Langman MJ. Audit of mortality in upper gastrointestinal bleeding. Postgraduate Medical Journal. 1989;**65**:913-917.

[8] Kerlin MP, Tokar JL. Acute gastrointestinal bleeding. Annals of Internal Medicine. 2013;**159**:793-794

[9] Palmer K. Management of haematemesis and melaena. Postgraduate Medical Journal 2004;**80**:399-404

[10] Barkun AN, Bardou M, Kuipers EJ, Sung J, Hunt RH, Martel M, et al. International consensus recommendations on the management of patients with nonvariceal upper gastrointestinal bleeding. Annals of Internal Medicine.2010;**152**:101-113

[11] Sung JJ, Chan FK, Chen M, Ching JY, Ho KY, Kachintorn U, et al. Asia-Pacific Working Group consensus on non-variceal upper gastrointestinal bleeding. Gut. 2011;**60**:1170-1177

[12] Gralnek IM, Dumonceau JM, Kuipers EJ, Lanas A, Sanders DS, Kurien M, et al. Diagnosis and management of nonvariceal upper gastrointestinal hemorrhage: European Society of Gastrointestinal Endoscopy (ESGE) Guideline. Endoscopy. 2015;**47**:a1-46

[13] Tripathi D, Stanley AJ, Hayes PC, Patch D, Millson C, Mehrzad H, et al. UK guidelines on the management of variceal haemorrhage in cirrhotic patients. Gut.2015;**64**:1680-1704

[14] de Franchis R. Expanding consensus in portal hypertension: Report of the Baveno VI Consensus Workshop: Stratifying risk and individualizing care for portal hypertension. Journal of Hepatology. 2015;**63**:743-752

[15] Garcia-Tsao G, Abraldes JG, Berzigotti A, Bosch J. Portal hypertensive bleeding in cirrhosis: Risk stratification, diagnosis, and management: 2016 practice guidance by the American Association for the study of liver diseases. Hepatology. 2017;**65**:310-335

[16] Hwang JH, Shergill AK, Acosta RD, Chandrasekhara V, Chathadi KV, Decker GA, et al. The role of endoscopy in the management of variceal hemorrhage. Gastrointestinal Endoscopy. 2014;**80**:221-227

[17] Hearnshaw S, Brunskill SJ, Doree C, Hyde C, Travis S, Murphy MF. Red cell transfusion for the management of upper gastrointestinal haemorrhage. The Cochrane Database of Systematic Reviews. 2009:CD006613

[18] Jairath V, Hearnshaw S, Brunskill SJ, Doree C, Hopewell S, Hyde C, et al. Red cell transfusion for the management of upper gastrointestinal haemorrhage. The Cochrane Database of Systematic Reviews. 2010:CD006613

[19] Wang J, Bao YX, Bai M, Zhang YG, Xu WD, Qi XS. Restrictive vs liberal transfusion for upper gastrointestinal bleeding: A meta-analysis of randomized controlled trials. World Journal of Gastroenterology. 2013;**19**:6919-6927

[20] Villanueva C, Colomo A, Bosch A, Concepcion M, Hernandez-Gea V, Aracil C, et al. Transfusion strategies for acute upper gastrointestinal bleeding. The New England Journal of Medicine. 2013;**368**:11-21

[21] Jairath V, Kahan BC, Gray A, Dore CJ, Mora A, James MW, et al. Restrictive versus liberal blood transfusion for acute upper gastrointestinal bleeding (TRIGGER): A pragmatic, open-label, cluster randomised feasibility trial. Lancet. 2015;**386**:137-144

[22] Jairath V, Kahan BC, Logan RF, Travis SP, Palmer KR, Murphy MF. Red blood cell transfusion practice in patients presenting with acute upper gastrointestinal bleeding: a survey of 815 UK clinicians. Transfusion. 2011;**51**:1940-1948

[23] Fortinsky KJ, Martel M, Razik R, Spiegle G, Gallinger ZR, Grover SC, et al. Red blood cell transfusions and iron therapy for patients presenting with acute upper gastrointestinal bleeding: A survey of Canadian gastroenterologists and hepatologists. Canadian Journal of Gastroenterology & Hepatology. 2016;**2016**:5610838